ORTHOPEDICS
Review & Self-Assessment

Kamal KV MBBS, MS (Orthopedics)
Ex-Senior Resident: Safdarjung, ESI – Okhla, Fortis – Noida
Ponseti and Ilizarov Techniques Fellow (Akola)
Madhya Pradesh – Indian Orthopedic Association
Hand Surgery Fellow (Pune), Maharashtra, India

Foreign (Academic) Trips (Countries and Cities)

Georgia (Tbilisi, Batumi)
Russia (Nalchik, Cheboksary, Stavropol, Kazan)
Kyrgyzstan (Jalalabad, Osh, Bishkek)
Nepal (Bharatpur, Bhairahawa, Dharan)
Ukraine (Vinnytsia, Kiev)
China (Ningbo, Nanchang, Nanning, Dali, Fuzhou, Guangzhou)
Belarus (Minsk)

For better results:

- Join drkamalkv's classes: The only not-for-profit classes
- Download drkamalkvgroup app from Google playstore (android)

Peepee Publishers and Distributors (P) Ltd.®

Orthopedics: Review and Self-Assessment

Published by
Pawaninder P. Vij and Anupam Vij

Peepee Publishers and Distributors (P) Ltd.
Head Office: 160, Shakti Vihar, Pitam Pura, Delhi-110 034 (India)

Correspondence Address:

7/31, First Floor, Ansari Road, Daryaganj
New Delhi-110 002 (India)

Ph: 41512412, 23246245, 9811156083

e-mail: peepee160@yahoo.co.in

e-mail: peepee160@gmail.com

www.peepeepub.com

join us on facebook.com/pp.publishers

First Edition: 2023

ISBN: 978-81-9523-446-2

DEDICATION

I would like to dedicate this title to all those who had arranged or served me during my foreign (academic) trips.

S. No.	*Countries*	*College*	*Timeline*
1.	**Georgia**	*i. Tbilisi*	Feb 2018
		ii. Batumi	Feb 2018
2.	**Russia**	*iii. Nalchik*	Oct 2018, Feb 2019, Dec 2019
		iv. Cheboksary	Oct 2018, Dec 2019
		v. Stavropol	Mar 2019
		vi. Kazan	Mar 2019
3.	**Kyrgyzstan**	*vii. Jalalabad*	Dec 2018, May 2019, Dec 2021, Dec 2022
		viii. Osh	May 2019, Dec 2022
		ix. Bishkek	Dec 2022
4.	**Nepal**	*x. Bhairahawa*	May 2019
		xi. Bharatpur	May 2019, Sep 2019
		xii. Dharan	Sep 2019
5.	**Ukraine**	*xiii. Vinnytsia*	Nov 2019
		xiv. Kiev	Nov 2019
6.	**China**	*xv. Ningbo*	Oct 2018
		xvi. Nanchang	Nov 2018
		xvii. Nanning	Nov 2018
		xviii. Dali	Nov 2018
		xix. Fuzhou	June 2019
		xx. Guangzhou	June 2019
7.	**Belarus**	*xxi. Minsk*	Jan 2020

PREFACE

There are many orthopedic books available in the market, but they are too bulky for the needs of NEET-PG/FMGE aspirants. A concise book covering all important examination topics was needed, so I have compiled the information to meet the students' needs. The book includes plenty of X-rays and images to aid in understanding.

As the name of the book is **Orthopedics: Review and Self-Assessment**, there are two main sections of the book:

1. **Review Notes:** Important text is arranged chapterwise, supported with related X-rays.
2. **Self-Assessment:** Questions are arranged in 3 sub-sections:
    - Image based MCQs.
    - Clinical MCQs.
    - MCQs points (simple and straightforward MCQs have been arranged as one-liner points for quick revision).

As I always say, students are the best judge of an author's work. I personally feel, there is always some room left for further improvement. So, I expect my dear students to share their valuable feedback regarding betterment of this text in subsequent editions.

Despite my best efforts, some errors must have crept in. I request dear readers to please forward the same to me.

Hope this title will serve its purpose.

31st January, 2023

drkamalkv

E-mail: **drkamalkvgroup**@gmail.com

Facebook/Telegram: **drkamalkvgroup**

WhatsApp: 84 7000 4333

ACKNOWLEDGEMENTS

As an Orthopedician, it was my dream (since long) to write a book on Orthopedics. But I was kept so much busy with other titles that I didn't got enough time to work on this project. I started writing books from 2009. Finally, after 13 years, this day has come, when I am writing this book on my specialty.

Let's discuss few basics of CTEV/clubfoot first.

One of the older method of CTEV corrective casting was **Kite's** method, which stressed that correct one deformity first before addressing the next deformity. Like first correct forefoot adductus, then hindfoot varus/inversion and finally equinus and the fulcrum was calcaneocuboid joint.

This technique is replaced nowadays by **Ponseti's** method where the fulcrum is head of the talus. Here cavus realignment is done by supinating the forefoot, then correct forefoot varus, inversion and adductus by abducting the foot beneath the stabilized head of the talus.

After his success, **Ponseti** quoted that it took so many years to shift the fingers (over fulcrum) from calcaneocuboid joint to head of talus. The same I can correlate that it took me 13 years to release a book of my own specialty. Anyway better late than never.

All thanks to Almighty (for imparting me with this passion of writing books and teaching), to my parents (for imparting qualities of a good human being), my brothers and sister (for giving me some wonderful memories of childhood), my wife (for supporting me in all my endeavours), my daughters (for allowing me to use their share of time with my students) and my dear students (for accepting my all titles with equal enthusiasm and also, who made me academically strong, to an extent).

Special thanks to **Mr. Pawaninder Paul Vij** and **Mr. Anupam Vij** for accepting all my work without any hesitancy or objection.

Thanks are due for everyone behind this project from the publication house.

drkamalkv

CONTENTS

SECTION 1

REVIEW NOTES

{CHAPTER WISE THEORY NOTES}

CHAPTER 1

INJURIES OF UPPER LIMB

FRACTURE CLAVICLE

Features

- Most commonly fractured bone in the body in all ages and gender.
- Most common site of fracture is the junction of medial 2/3rd and lateral 1/3rd.
- Managed by figure of 8 bandage.
- Fracture unites readily even if widely displaced.
- Most common complication is malunion.

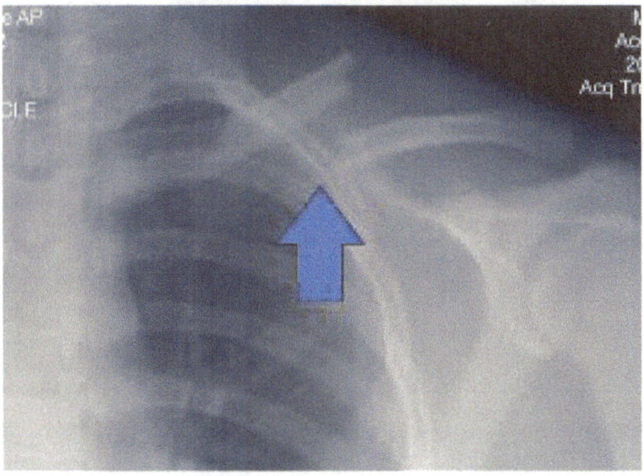

FRACTURE SCAPULA

Features

- Uncommon and unimportant.
- Patient recover well without much treatment.
- Fracture fragments are held in place by the surrounding muscles so fracture heals well with a triangular sling.

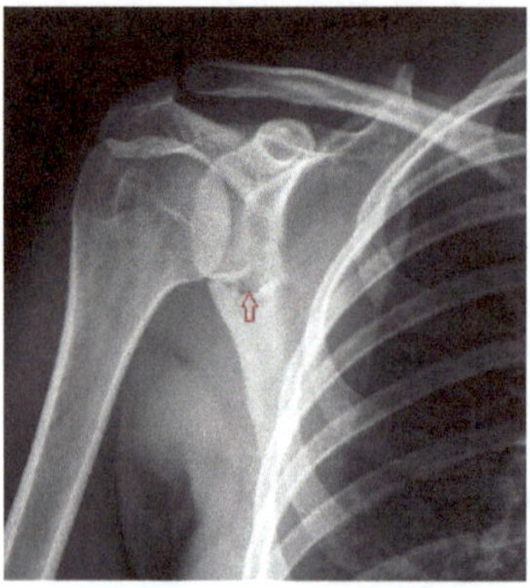

FRACTURE SURGICAL NECK OF HUMERUS

Features

- **Axillary nerve** can get injured resulting in atrophy of the deltoid muscle and regiment badge sign.

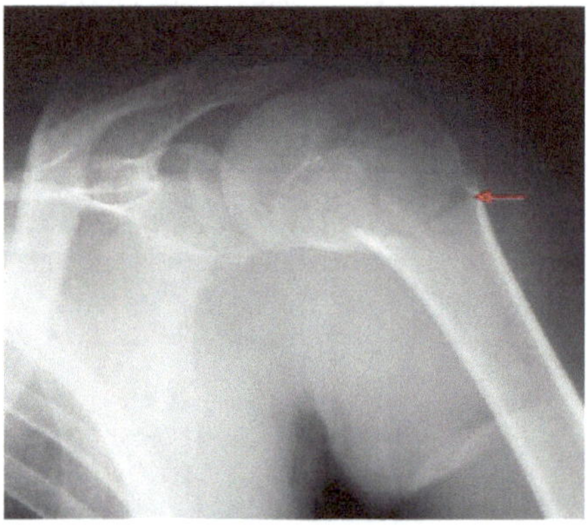

DISLOCATION OF SHOULDER JOINT

Features

- Shoulder joint is the **most common (MC)** joint to dislocate.
- Shoulder joint is the **most common** joint to undergo recurrent dislocation.
- **Most common** mechanism of injury is FOOSH (**F**all **O**n **O**ut **S**tretched **H**and) with shoulder externally rotated.
- **Most common** type: Sub-coracoid type (Anterior dislocation).

- Luxatio erecta: Head of humerus lies in subglenoid region.
- **Rare** type: Posterior dislocation (associated with epilepsy or electric shock).
- *Clinical tests:*
  - Dugas test: Patient is unable to touch the opposite shoulder.
  - Callaway's test: There is an increase in vertical circumference of axilla as compared to opposite side.
  - Hamilton ruler's test: Normally one cannot put a ruler on the lateral aspect of arm touching the acromion and lateral condyle of humerus simultaneously but in anterior dislocation, because of shoulder flattening, ruler will touch both the anatomical landmarks simultaneously.
- *Management:*
  - Managed by closed reduction by Kocher's manoeuvre.
  - Steps are **TEAM** (**T**raction, **E**xternal rotation, **A**dduction and **M**edial/internal rotation).
- *Complications:*
  - Axillary nerve damage and
  - Recurrent dislocation.
- *Recurrent dislocation shows:*
  - Bankart's lesion (glenoidal labrum).
  - Hill Sach's lesion (humeral lesion).

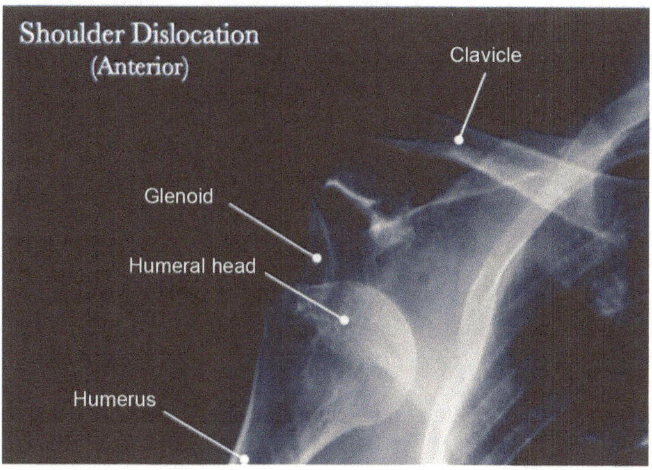

ROTATOR CUFF MUSCLES

Features

- *Muscles in rotator cuff* ***(Mnemonic: SITS)****:*
    - **S**upraspinatus.
    - **I**nfraspinatus.
    - **T**eres minor.
    - **S**ubscapularis.
- Rotator interval is between: Supraspinatus and subscapularis.
- Most commonly damaged muscle in rotator cuff: Supraspinatus.

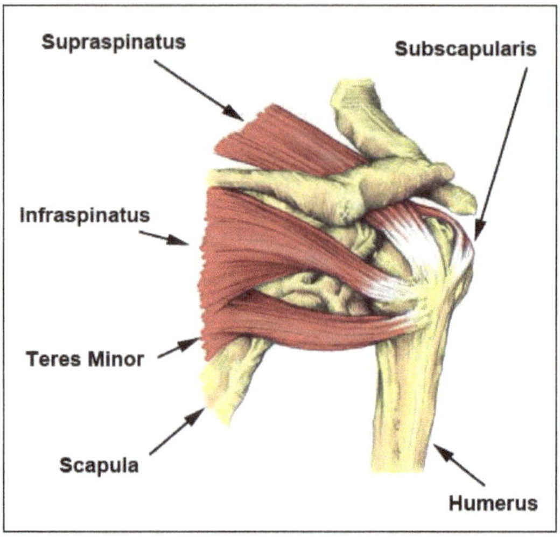

FRACTURE SHAFT OF HUMERUS

Features

- **Lateral angulation** is common because of abduction of proximal fragment by deltoid muscle.
- **Radial nerve** can be injured resulting in wrist drop (Radial nerve passes through spiral/ radial groove).
- Managed by U-slab, **hanging cast**.
- Union occurs early because of abundant blood supply.
- Some degree of malunion is acceptable due to thick muscle cover all around.

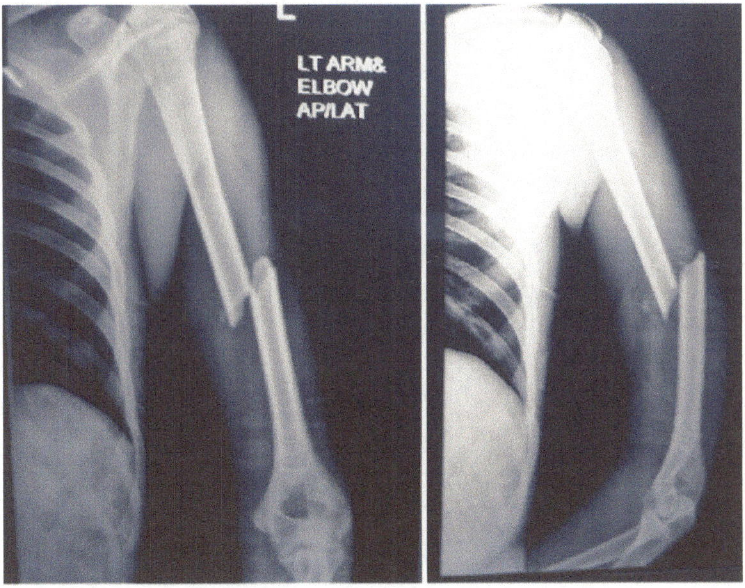

FRACTURE SUPRACONDYLAR HUMERUS

Features

- Commonly seen in **children** (not seen in adults).
- **Most common** type: Extension.
- 3-point bony relationship is **maintained** at elbow.
- Displaced fractures are managed by closed reduction and plaster or open reduction and **K-wire** fixation.
- Fracture fragment can cause injury to brachial artery which may cause **Volkmann's ischemia** (ischemia of forearm muscles).
- Untreated Volkmann's ischemia may result in in Volkmann's ischemic contracture.
- Malunion is the **most common** complication leading to **cubitus varus/ gun stock deformity**.
- Myositis ossificans.
- **Median nerve** (or more commonly anterior interosseous nerve) injury.

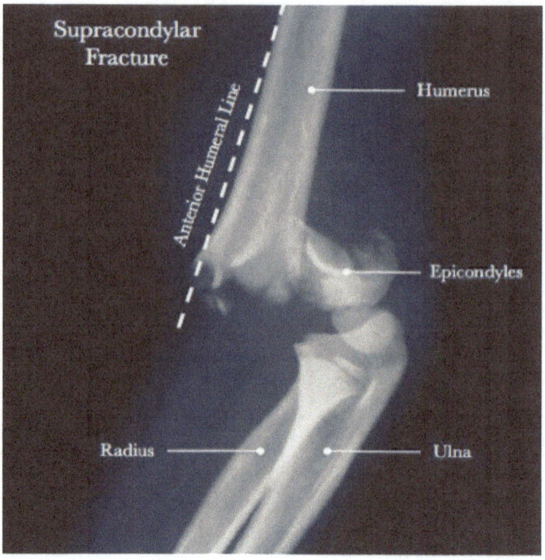

FRACTURE LATERAL CONDYLE OF HUMERUS

Features

- **Accurate reduction** is very important for normal growth of elbow.
- Therefore, this fracture is managed by open reduction and internal fixation by K-wires (right side image).
- Neglected cases develop **cubitus valgus** deformity which can later on cause ulnar nerve palsy (**Tardy ulnar nerve palsy**).

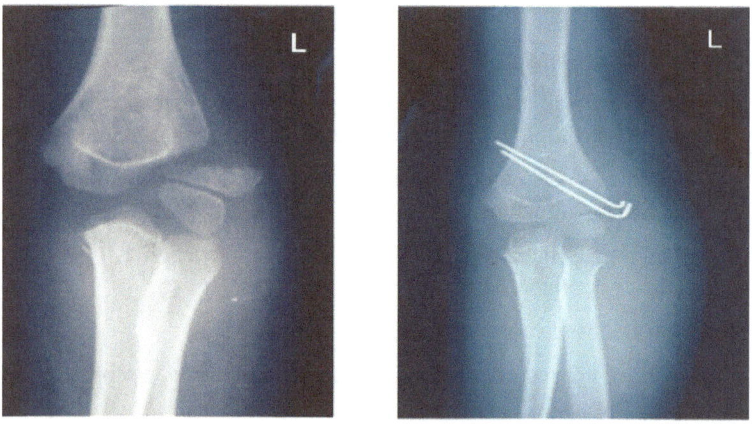

POSTERIOR DISLOCATION OF ELBOW

Features

- 3-point bony relationship is **disturbed** (between medial epicondyle, lateral epicondyle and tip of olecranon process).
- Can cause ulnar nerve injury.

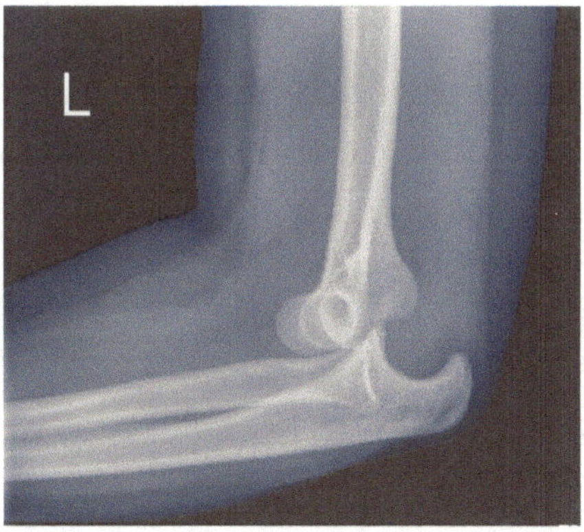

PULLED ELBOW

Features

- Also known as Nurse maid's elbow.
- There is subluxation of radial head from annular ligament/ Subluxation of the annular ligament which slips over the head of radius.
- Occurs due to sudden **axial pull** on extended elbow.
- Forearm in held in pronation and extension.
- X-rays are **normal**.
- Treatment is reduction by flexing the elbow to 90 degrees and rotating the forearm into full supination.

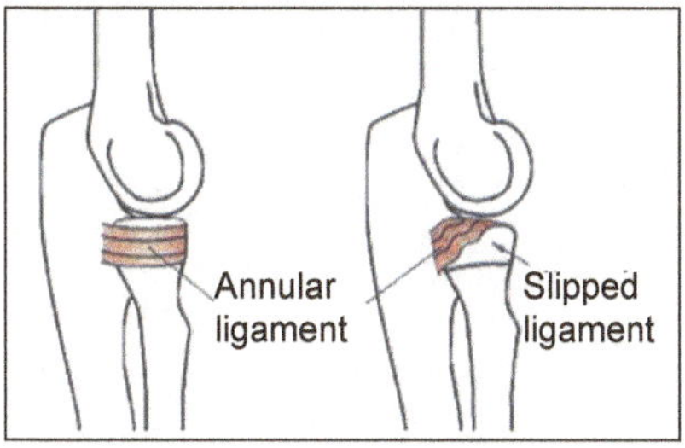

FRACTURE RADIAL HEAD

Features

- Mason classification is used.
- Essex Lopresti fracture: Fracture radial head + injury to interosseous membrane.
- *Management:*
  - In adults, head of the radius, if fractured, can be excised.
  - Excision of head of radius will cause cubitus valgus deformity.
  - Excision of radial head in a child should **NOT** be done as it causes subluxation of inferior radio-ulnar joint.

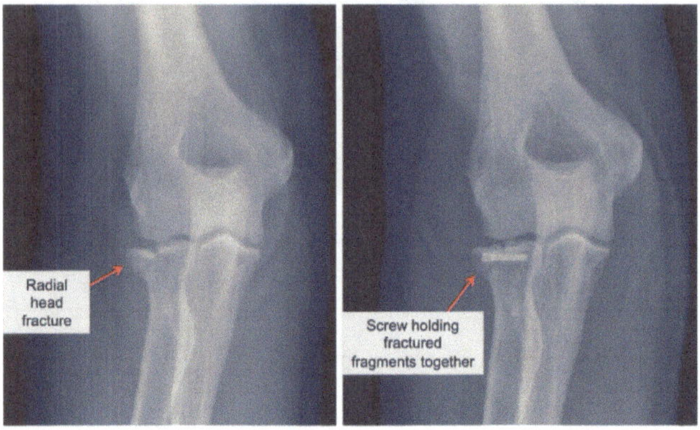

FRACTURE OLECRANON PROCESS

Features

- Occurs due to fall on point of elbow.
- Displaced fractures are managed by **Tension Band Wiring** (TBW).

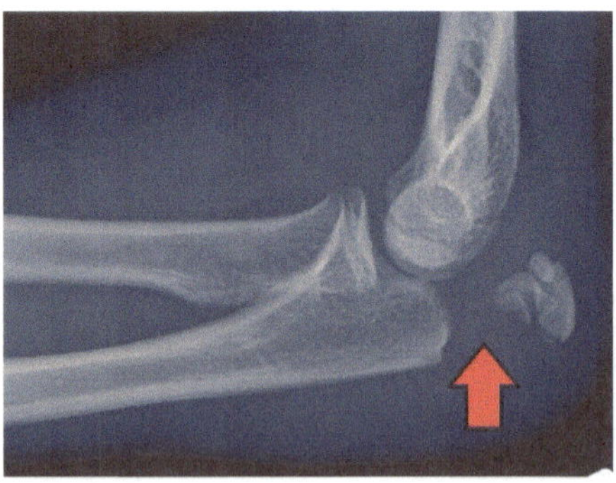

FRACTURE BOTH BONE FOREARM

Features

- One of the common injuries of childhood.
- In children, closed reduction and plaster of Paris cast is enough.
- In adults, open reduction and internal fixation by plates is usually done.
- Volkmann's ischemia may occur.

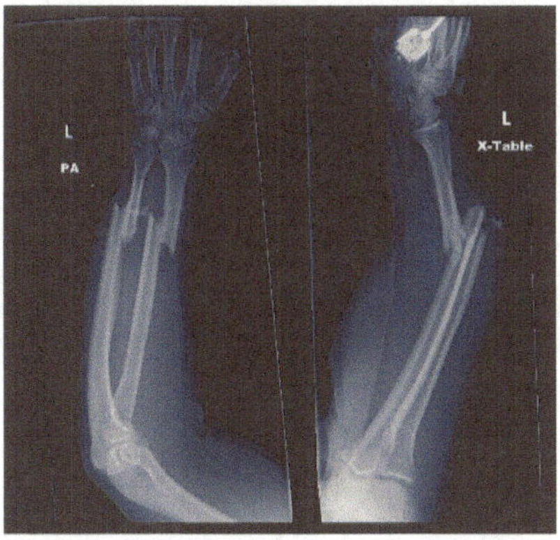

MONTEGGIA FRACTURE DISLOCATION

Features

- Fracture of proximal third of ulna + Dislocation of proximal radio-ulnar joint.
- Extension type is commoner.
- Both ulnar fracture and head of radius is displaced anteriorly.
- Posterior interosseous nerve can be injured (result in paralysis of thumb and finger extensors).

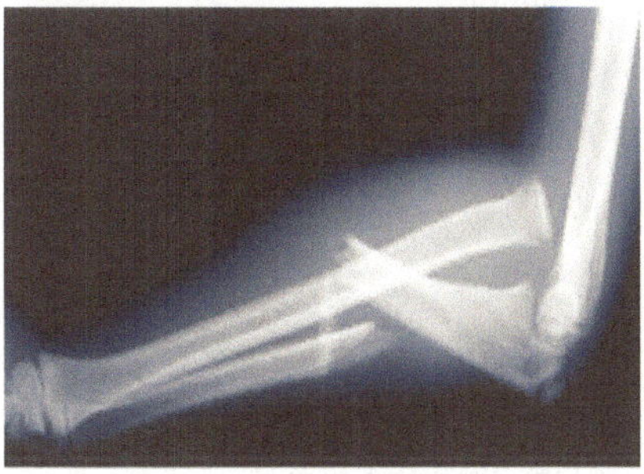

GALEAZZI FRACTURE-DISLOCATION

Features

- Fracture of the distal third of the shaft of **radius** + Dislocation of the **distal** radio-ulnar joint.

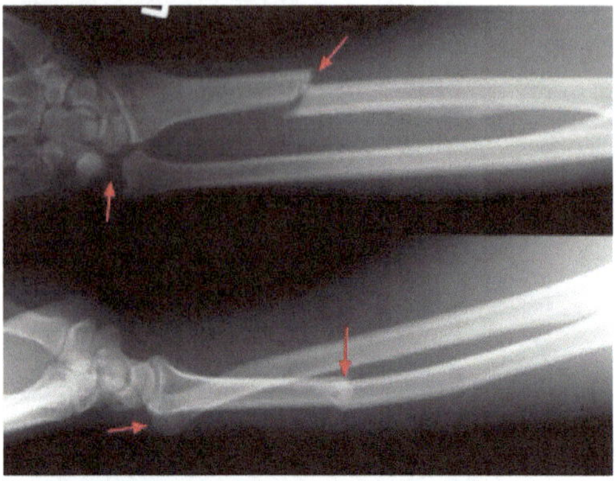

FRACTURE COLLE'S

Features

- Fracture occurs at the cortico-cancellous junction of the **lower end of radius**.
- Usually seen in **elderly post-menopausal women** are at risk (because of osteoporosis).
- Normally radial styloid process is at a lower level than ulnar styloid process, but in Colle's fracture, radial styloid process comes to lie at the same level or at a higher level than ulnar styloid process.
- *6 characteristic movements of distal fragment:*
    - Lateral shift.
    - Lateral angulation.
    - Dorsal shift.
    - Dorsal angulation (see image).
    - Supination.
    - Impaction.
- Characteristic deformity: **Dinner fork deformity**.
- Patient is managed by closed reduction and application of cast (in palmar flexion and ulnar deviation).

- Finger stiffness is the **most common** complication.

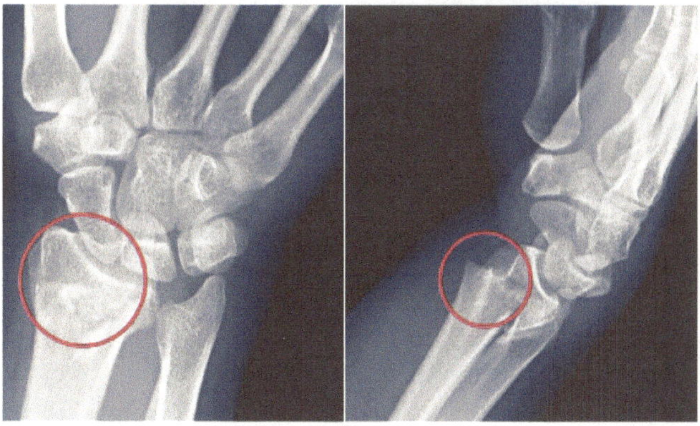

FRACTURE SMITH'S

Features

- Also known as **reverse** Colle's fracture.
- Garden spade deformity.

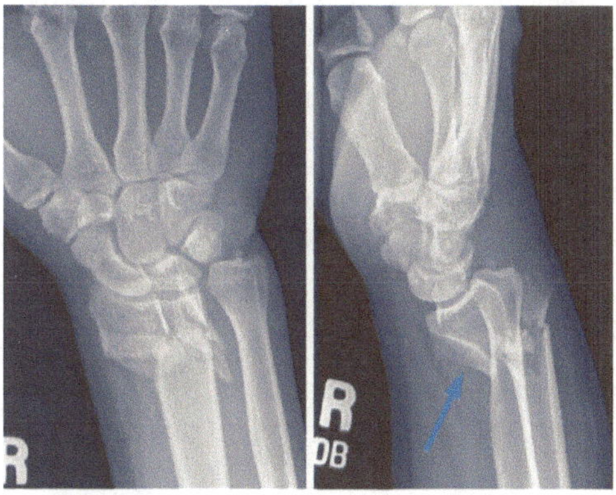

FRACTURE BARTON'S

Features

- A fracture-dislocation in which the carpus and a rim of distal radius are displaced together.
- Depending on the displacement, there can be volar or dorsal Barton fracture.

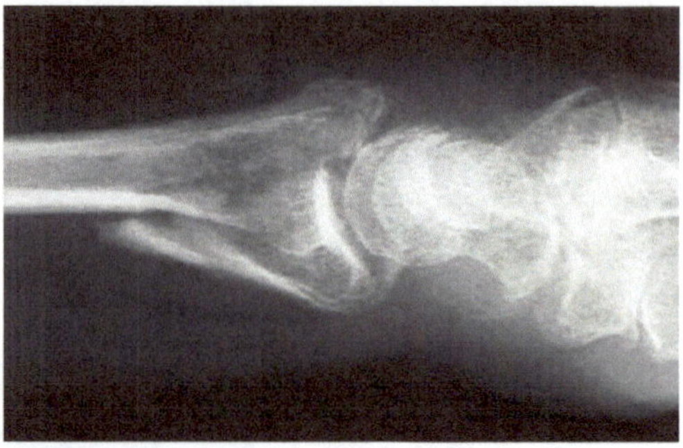

FRACTURE SCAPHOID

Features

- Scaphoid is the only carpal bone to undergo fracture as well as AVN/ **avascular necrosis**.
- Fragment undergoing necrosis in fracture scaphoid: **Proximal**.
- **Most common** site of fracture scaphoid: Waist.
- Clinically patient comes with pain and **tenderness over anatomical snuff box** after a **FOOSH** (**F**all **O**n **O**ut**S**tretched **H**and).
- Anatomical snuff box lies between tendons of EPL (extensor pollicis longus) and EPB (extensor pollicis brevis).
- Initial X-rays does **NOT** show fracture and hence diagnosis is always clinical.
- Oblique views should be done at the time of injury and after 2 weeks to look for fracture line.
- Managed by scaphoid cast application in **glass holding position**.

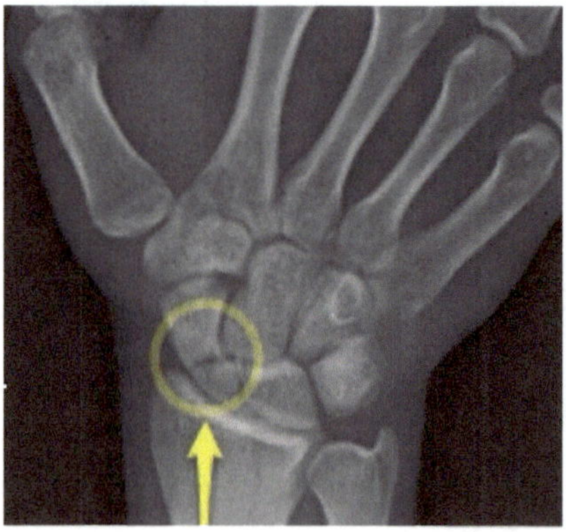

LUNATE DISLOCATION

Features

- Lunate dislocates anteriorly.
- Rest of the carpal remains in position.

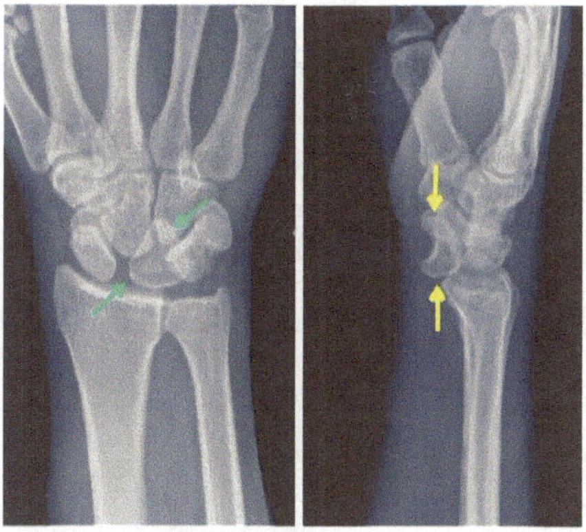

PERILUNATE DISLOCATION

Features

- Lunate remains in position.
- Rest of the carpals dislocates dorsally.
- **More common** type of injury.
- Median nerve is **commonly** injured.

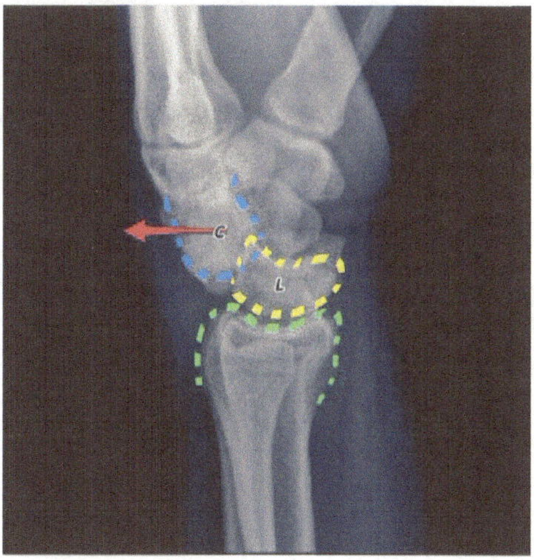

FRACTURE BENNET'S

Features

- Intra-articular fracture through the base of 1st metacarpal.
- Shaft is laterally dislocated because of unopposed pull of the abductor pollicis longus.

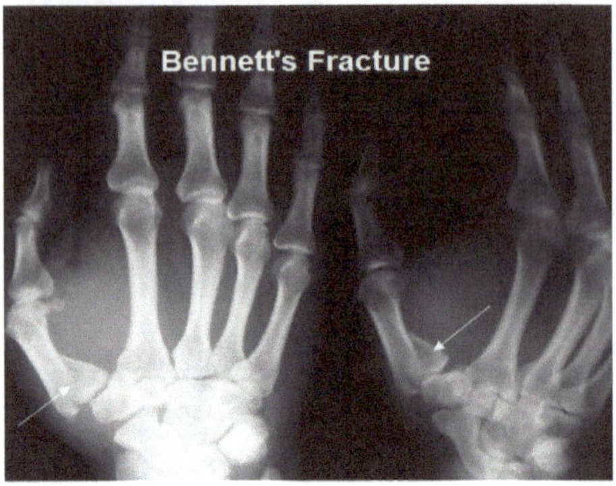

FRACTURE ROLANDO

Features

- T or Y-shaped intra-articular fracture involving the base of 1st metacarpal.

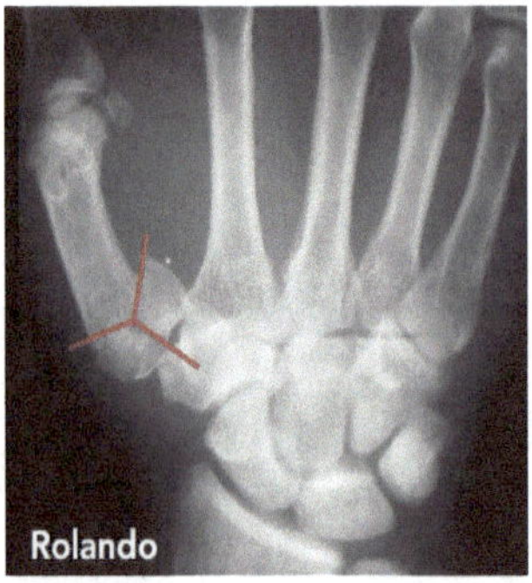

CHAPTER 2

INJURIES OF LOWER LIMB

FRACTURE PELVIS

Features

- Occurs in vehicular injuries.
- In cases of isolated fractures, ischiopubic rami is **most commonly** fractured.
- Iliac wings are very vascular so importance should be given in managing **hypovolemic shock** first.
- *Complications:*
    - Rupture of membranous urethra.
    - Extra-peritoneal rupture of bladder with extravasation of urine into peri-vesical space.

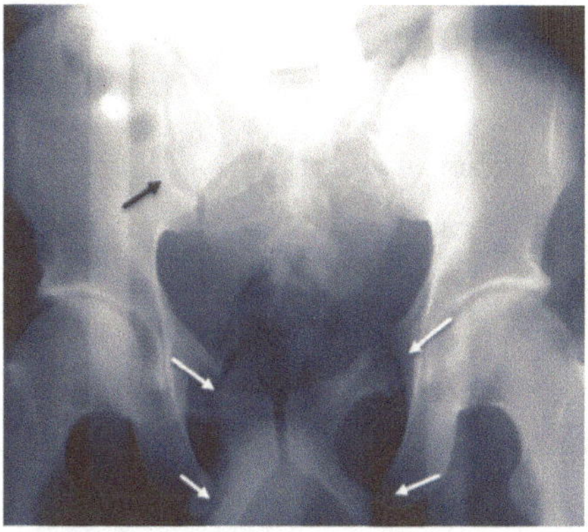

FRACTURE ACETABULUM

Features

- Judet view (X-ray) is taken.
- Spur sign is seen on X-ray.

- *Complications:*
  - Sciatic nerve injury.
  - AVN of femoral head.
  - Secondary osteoarthritis of the hip joint.

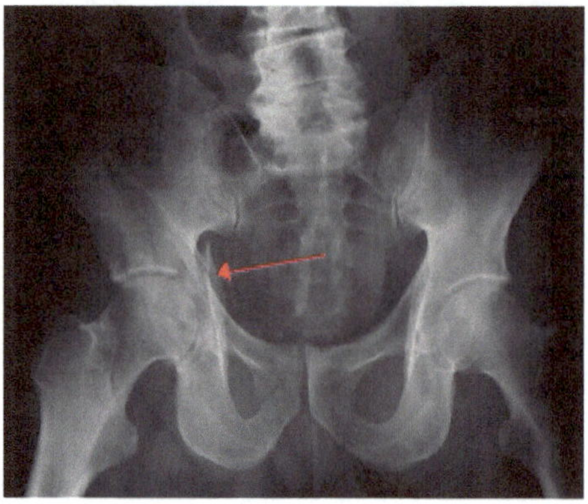

POSTERIOR HIP DISLOCATION

Features

- Most common type of hip dislocation: Posterior dislocation.
- *Attitude of limb in posterior hip dislocation is **FADIR**:*
  - **F**lexion.
  - **Ad**duction.
  - **I**nternal **R**otation.
- Posterior hip dislocation commonly occurs because of dashboard injury (car).
- *X-ray:*
  - Broken Shenton line.
  - Shenton line is a continuous curved line formed by neck of femur and inferior border of superior pubic rami.
- *Emergency reduction needs to be done:*
  - Stimpson's gravity.
  - Allis manoeuvre.
- Can injure sciatic nerve.

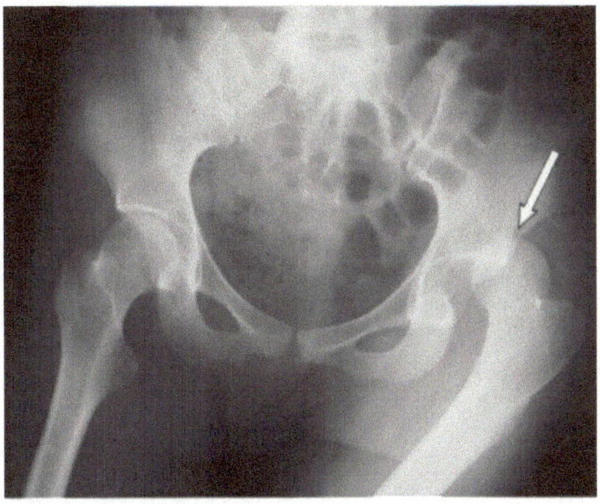

ANTERIOR HIP DISLOCATION

Features

- Occurs when the hip is externally rotated and abducted.
- *Attitude of limb in anterior hip dislocation is **FABER**:*
    - **F**lexion.
    - **Ab**duction.
    - **E**xternal **R**otation.
- Associated with lengthening.

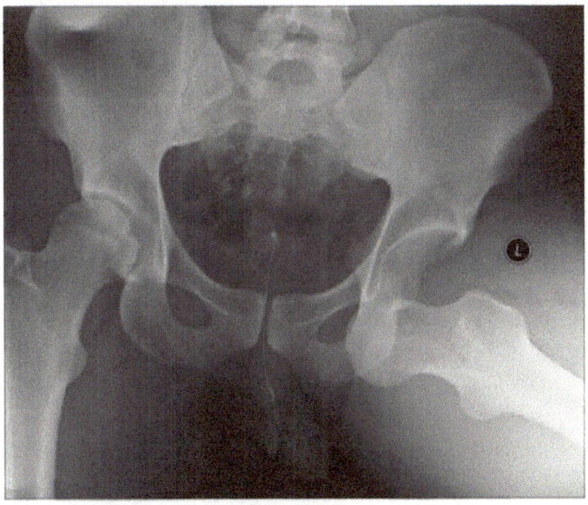

CENTRAL HIP DISLOCATION

Features

- Femoral head is forced medially through the floor of acetabulum.
- Head of femur can be palpated on per-rectal examination.

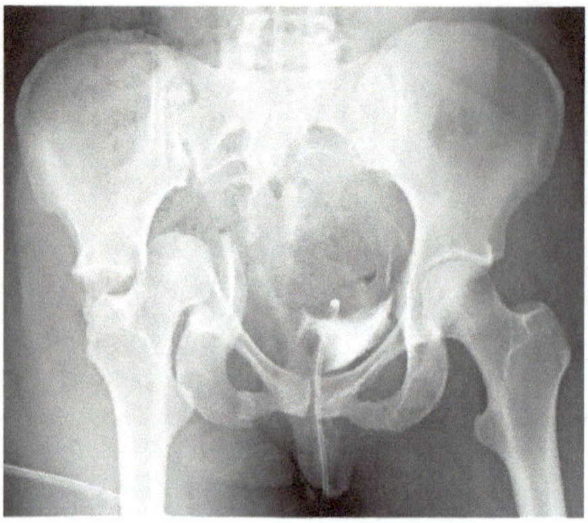

FRACTURE NECK OF FEMUR (INTRA-CAPSULAR)

Features

- *Classification:*
  - Anatomical.
  - Pauwel's.
  - Garden's.
- *Mechanism:*
  - Occurs in **elderly** after a trivial fall.
  - Osteoporosis is considered as an important factor.
- *Diagnosis:*
  - External rotation of leg.
  - **Shortening** of leg.
  - Movements of hip are painful.
  - Active straight leg raising is not possible.
- *X-ray:*
  - Break in medial cortex of the neck.
  - **External rotation** of the femur is evident.
  - Over-riding of greater trochanter, so that it lies at the level of the head of femur.
  - Break in **Shenton's** line.
  - Break in the tubercular stream.

- *Treatment:*
  - Internal fixation:
    - Multiple cancellous screws.
    - Dynamic hip screw.
    - Multiple Knowle's pins/Moore's pin (in children).
  - McMurray's osteotomy.
  - Hemiarthroplasty in **elderly** (above 60 years of age).
  - Meyer's procedure.
- *Complications:*
  - **Non-union**.
  - **Avascular necrosis**.
  - Osteoarthritis.

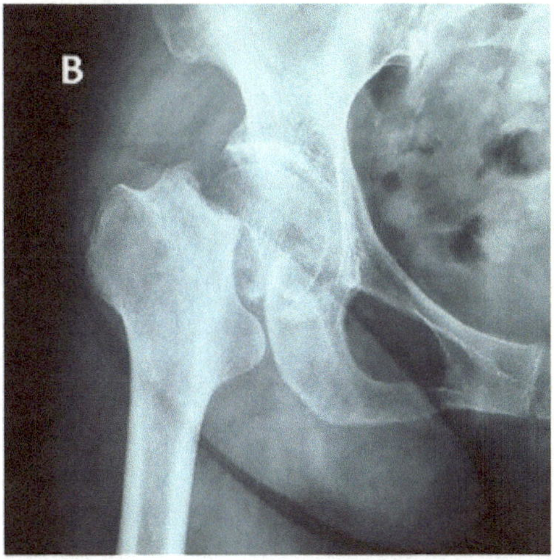

FRACTURE NECK OF FEMUR (EXTRA-CAPSULAR)

Features

- Also known as intertrochanteric fracture.
- Swelling and ecchymosis over greater trochanter with broadening of greater trochanter.
- External rotation of lower limb is more than 45 degrees.
- Managed by proximal femoral nail and DHS.

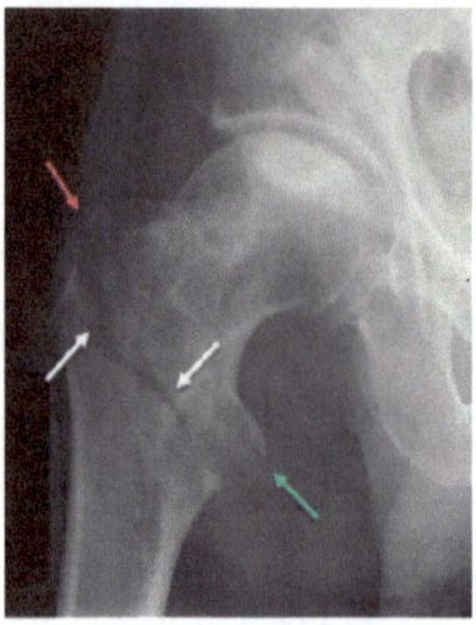

FRACTURE SUB-TROCHANTER FEMUR

Features

- Managed by cephalon-medullary nail.

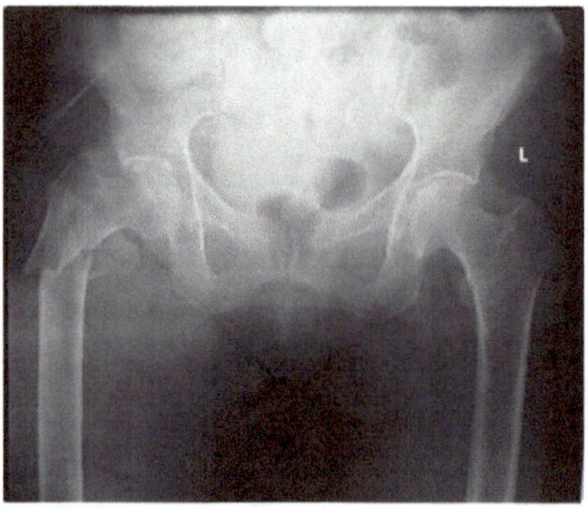

FRACTURE SHAFT OF FEMUR

Features

- Usually occurs because of high velocity Road Traffic Accident
- May lead to **hypovolemic shock** (because of excess blood loss) and fat **embolism**
- In adults, managed operatively by interlock nailing
- *Management of fracture shaft of femur in children:*
    - Gallows traction: <2 years
    - Hip spica: 2-5 years
    - Ender's nail: >6 years

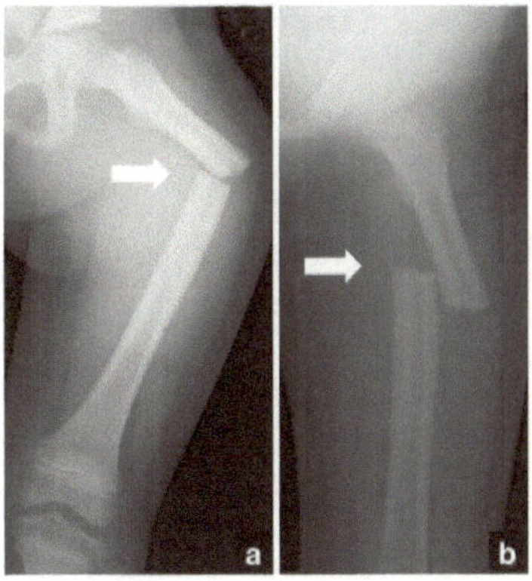

FRACTURE PATELLA

Features

- *May result from:*
  - Direct force (causing stellate or comminuted fracture).
  - Indirect force (causing **2-part** fracture).
- Patient presents with pain and swelling over knee joint.
- There is **extensor lag** (patient is unable to lift leg with the knee in full extension).
- *X-ray views:* AP, lateral and sometime **skyline view**.
- *Management:*
  - Un-displaced fracture: POP cast with knee in extension.
  - Displaced fracture: Tension Band Wiring/**TBW** with K-wires and stainless-steel wires.
  - Comminuted fractures: Patellectomy.

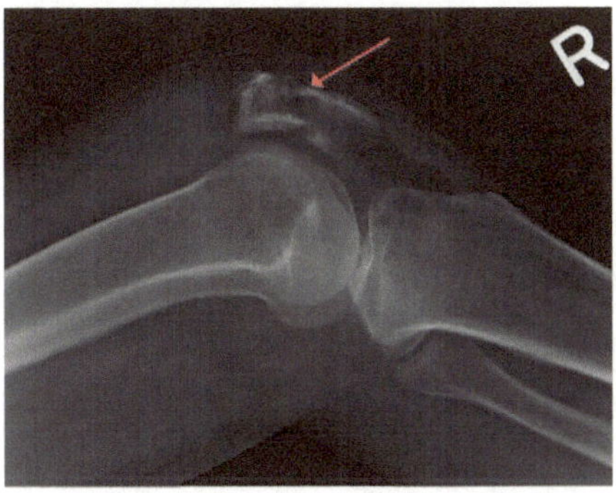

COLLATERAL LIGAMENT INJURY

Features

- *Medial collateral ligament injury:*
  - Valgus force over the knee injures medial collateral ligament.
  - Tested by valgus/abduction stress test in 30 degrees of knee flexion.
- *Lateral collateral ligament injury:*
  - Varus force over the knee injures lateral collateral ligament.
  - Tested by varus/adduction stress test in 30 degrees of knee flexion.
- Treatment is reconstruction.

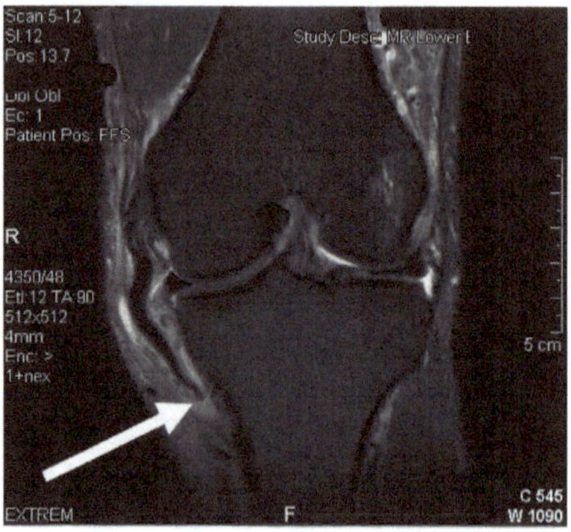

ANTERIOR CRUCIATE LIGAMENT INJURY

Features

- **Most commonly** injured ligament of knee joint.
- Prevents anterior translation of the tibia on femur.
- *Clinical **test** for ACL tear:*
  - Lachman test
  - Anterior drawer test
- Presents with popping sound and patient feel knee instability or **giving away** of knee joint.
- **MRI** is the investigation of choice.

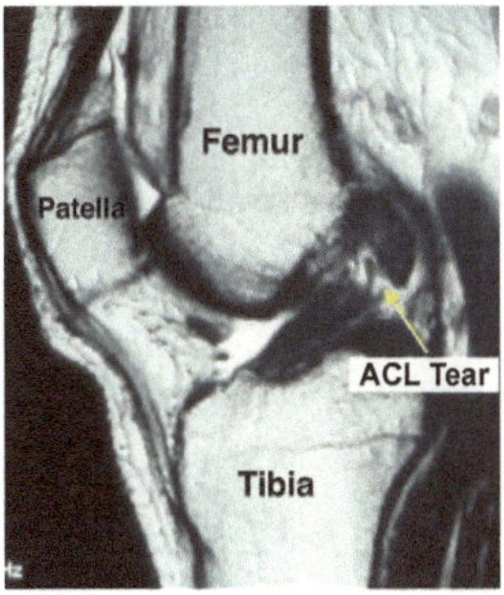

MEDIAL MENISCUS TEAR

Features

- Medial meniscus is injured **more commonly** than lateral meniscus as it is less mobile.
- *Clinical test for medial meniscus tear:*
  - McMurray test.
  - Apley's grinding test.
- *O'Donoghue unhappy triad:*
  - Medial collateral ligament tear.
  - ACL tear.
  - Medial meniscus tear.
- **MRI** is the investigation of choice.

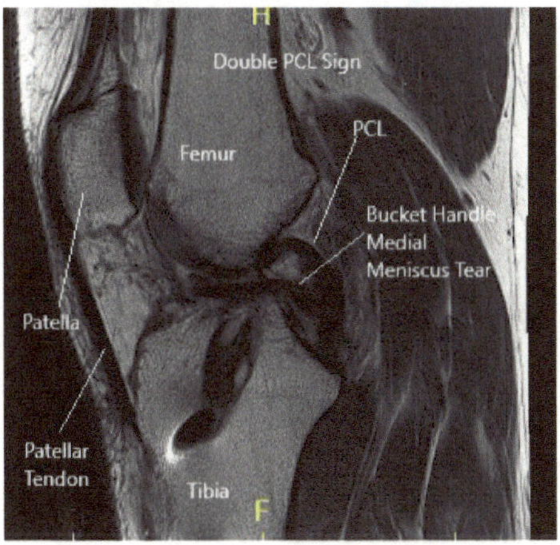

FRACTURE TIBIA-FIBULA

Features

- Fractures in the lower one-third go into delayed-union or **non-union** as blood supply is precarious.
- *Management:*
  - Children: Plaster of Paris cast.
  - Adults:
    - Open Reduction and Internal Fixation (**ORIF**) with plate and screws.
    - Closed Reduction and Internal Fixation (CRIF) with interlock nailing.

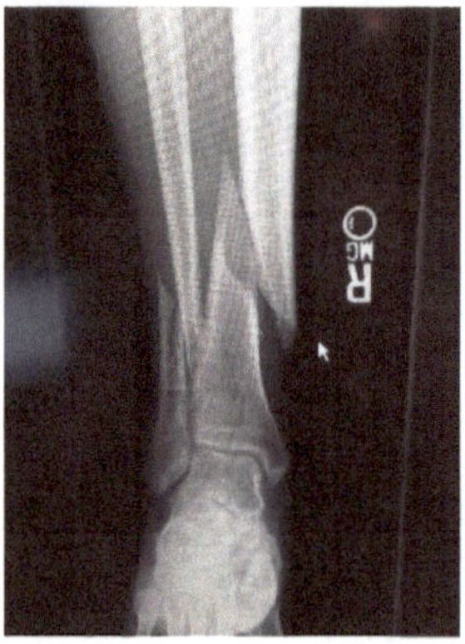

ANKLE INJURIES

Features

- *Lauge-Hansen classification of ankle fractures:*
  - Supination-inversion injury.
  - Supination-external rotation injury.
  - Pronation-abduction injury.
  - Pronation-external rotation injury.
- *Fractures involving malleoli:*
  - Pott's fracture:
    - Bimalleolar.
    - Medial and lateral malleolus.

- Cotton's fracture:
  - Trimalleolar.
  - Medial, lateral and posterior malleolus.

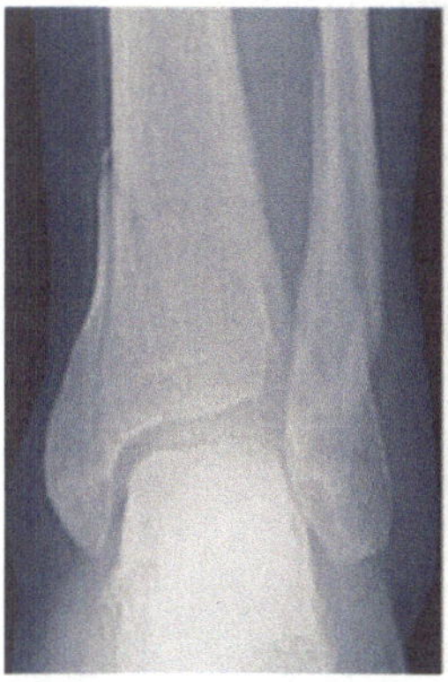

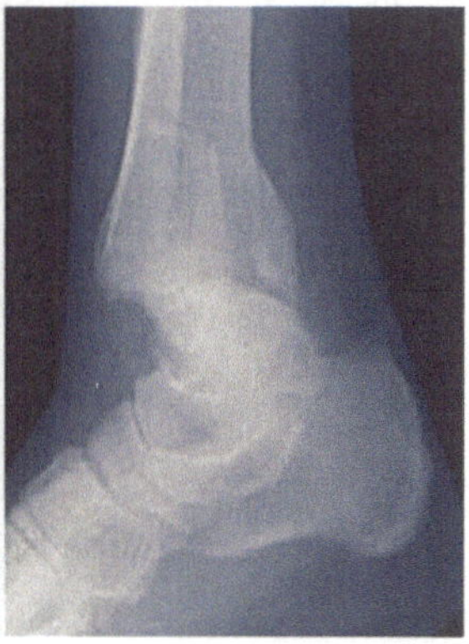

FRACTURE NECK OF TALUS

Features

- Also known as aviator's fracture.
- Usually seen in pilots, who jump from the plane.
- Common complication is avascular necrosis.
- *Hawkin's sign:*
  - If positive, indicates a good prognosis (good vascularity of talus).
  - It indicates viability at 6-8 weeks after fracture.
  - It is a subchondral radio-lucent band in the talar dome.

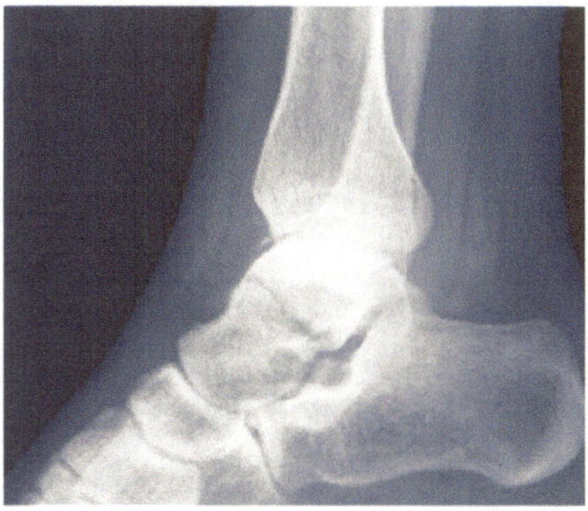

FRACTURE CALCANEUM

Features

- Usually due to fall from **height** onto the heels.
- May be **associated** with fractures of lumbar spine.
- Best seen on lateral X-ray of foot.

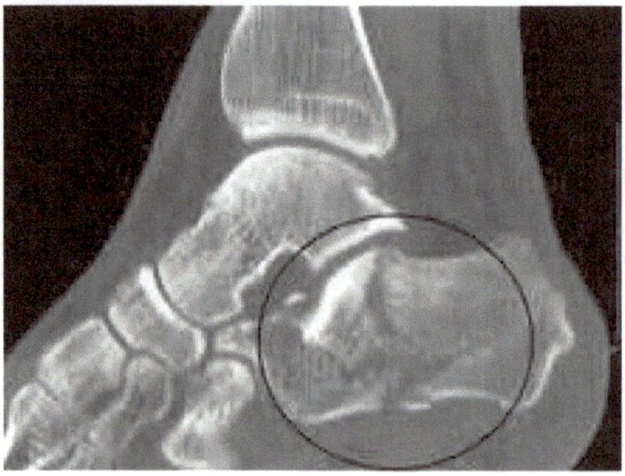

CHAPTER 3

INFECTIONS OF BONE AND JOINTS

ACUTE OSTEOMYELITIS/ OM

Features

- **Earliest** site of involvement in primary OM:
  - Metaphysis.
  - Because metaphysis is the growing highly vascular region of bone with hair-pin arrangement of vessels.
- **Most common** organism in acute OM: Staphylococcus aureus (In **sickle cell** anemia patients, OM is usually caused by salmonella).
- **Most common** site of acute OM in children: Lower femoral epiphysis.
- **Most common** type of osteomyelitis: Secondary accounts for 80% cases (from contiguous focus of infection because of open/ compound fractures or bony operative procedures which get infected).
- In children, **most common** type is primary, which is hematogenous in origin.
- Diagnosis of acute OM is always clinical.
- **Diagnosis** of acute OM: Blood culture (positive in 65% cases).
- *X-ray:*
  - Early X-ray may be normal.
  - **Periosteal reaction** (periosteal new bone formation) seen in acute OM appears after: 10 days (therefore bony changes are not supportive in making a diagnosis of acute OM).
- Bone scan show increased uptake.

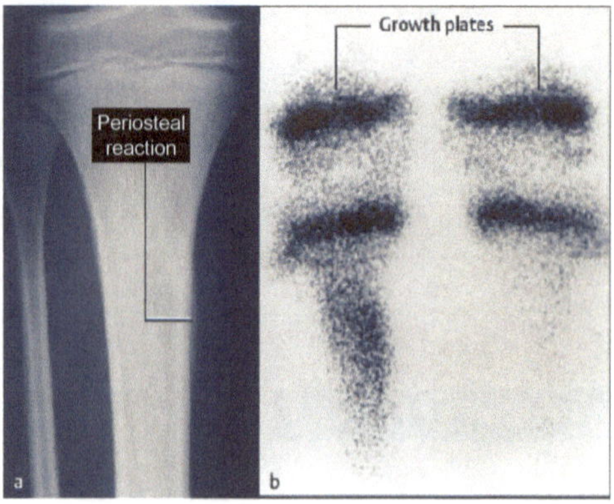

- MRI may show changes within 48 hours and is the IOC.
- Management is with broad spectrum antibiotics if the patient reports within 48 hours. Otherwise, it is presumed that pus has formed and surgical exploration and drainage is needed.
- MC complication of acute OM is chronic OM.
- *Other complications:*
    - Pathological fracture.
    - Acute pyogenic arthritis (if metaphysis is intra-articular).
    - Growth plate disturbances.

CHRONIC OSTEOMYELITIS

Features

- Chronic OM is the **most common** complication of untreated/ inadequately treated OM.
- **Most common** site is lower end of femur.
- **Most common** presenting symptom is chronic discharging sinus.
- *Clinical presentation:*
    - Discharge of bony spicules through the sinus is almost **diagnostic** of chronic osteomyelitis.
    - Thickened irregular bone.
    - Tenderness.
    - Stiffness of adjacent joints.
- *X-ray:*

- **Sequestrum** is defined as dead-piece of bone surrounded by infected granulation tissue.
- **Involucrum** is defined as dense sclerotic bone overlying sequestrum.
- **Cloacae** are the opening in bones through which necrotic matter is discharged.

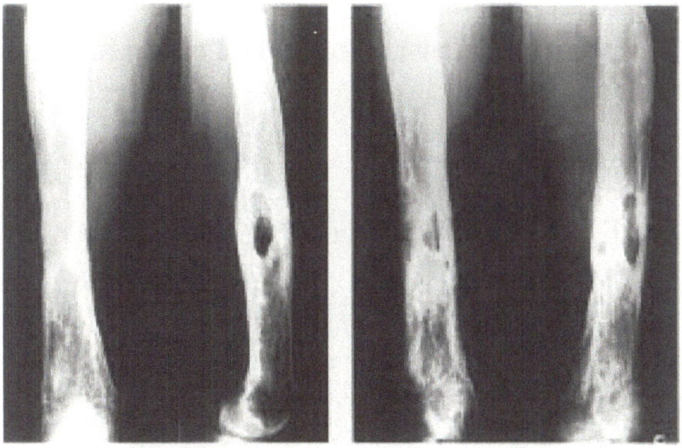

- *Always require surgical treatment:*
  - Sequestrectomy.
  - Saucerization.
  - Curettage.
  - Excision (fibula).
  - After surgery, a continuous suction irrigation system is done.
- *Complications:*
  - Acute exacerbations/Flare up.
  - Growth abnormalities.
  - Pathological fracture.
  - Stiffness of joints.
  - Sinus tract malignancy.
  - Amyloidosis.

BRODIE'S ABSCESS

Features

- Subacute osteomyelitis.

- Equilibrium between host & organism.
- Abscess cavity remains without further enlargement.
- A type of chronic bone abscess.
- Contains pus/jelly like granulation tissue surrounded by a zone of sclerosis.
- *X-ray:*
    - Oval/ circular lucent area surrounded by zone of sclerosis.

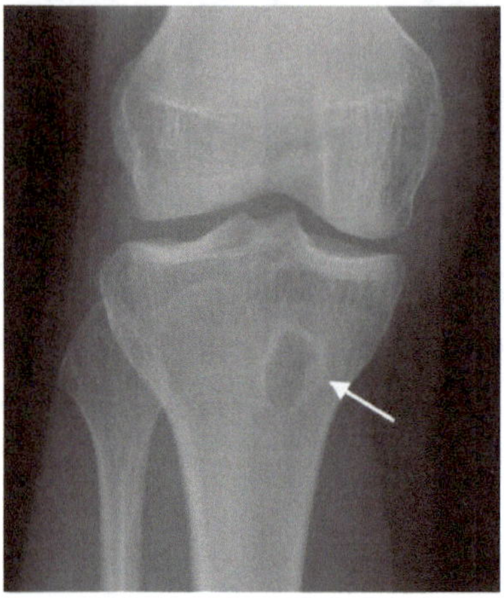

GARRE'S OSTEOMYELITIS

Features

- It is a type of chronic OM which is sclerosing, non-suppurative and without any discharging sinus.

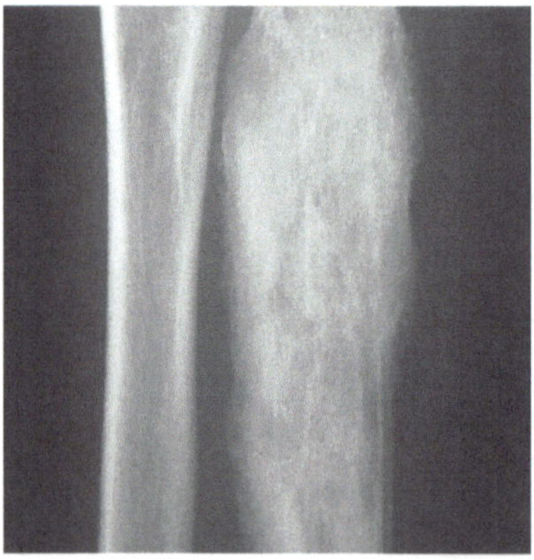

SEPTIC ARTHRITIS

Features

- Seen more commonly in children.
- MC (most common) caused by staphylococcus aureus.
- MC route is hematogenous.
- May be a complication of nearby osteomyelitis.
- *Clinical presentation:*
    - Severe throbbing pain.
    - Swelling.
    - Redness of the affected joint.
    - High grade fever.
- *Diagnosis:*
    - Joint aspiration:
        - Quickest and best method.
        - Synovial fluid findings of acute septic arthritis:
            - WBC count: >10,000 (normally <200).
            - Neutrophils > 75% (normally <25%).
            - Culture is positive.
            - Glucose level is more than 25% of blood glucose.
    - Blood:
        - Neutrophilic leucocytosis.
        - Blood culture may grow the causative organism.
    - X-ray:
        - Normal in early stages.
        - One may be seen increased joint space.
- *Treatment:*
    - Start broad spectrum antibiotics.
    - Do joint aspiration; if pus comes out then do arthrotomy. Give a wash and closed the joint over suction drain.
    - In late cases, with joint damage, do arthrotomy, joint debridement and immobilization in optimum position to allow

ankylosis in that position (like knee should be immobilized in flexion, wrist in dorsiflexion etc.).

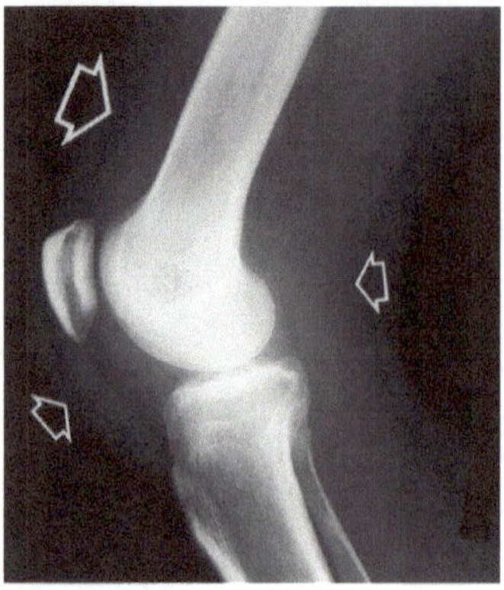

TOM SMITHS ARTHRITIS

Features

- Septic arthritis of infancy.
- Head of femur is cartilaginous so it is completely destroyed by the septic process.

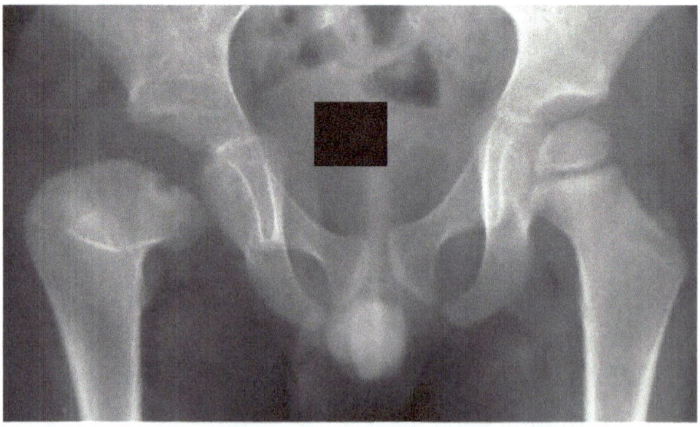

MUSCULOSKELETAL TUBERCULOSIS/ MSTB

Features

- TB in body:
  - Lungs.
  - LN.
  - Musculoskeletal system.

- Musculoskeletal TB is always secondary.
- *Outcome of healed MSTB is ankylosis:*
  - *Bony ankylosis:* TB spine.
  - *Fibrous ankylosis:* Other joints.
- Causes slow destruction (unlike pyogenic arthritis)
- Systemic symptoms (fever, loss of appetite, loss of weight) are less marked
- *X-ray:*
  - Reduction of joint space.
  - Erosion of articular surfaces.
  - Periarticular rarefaction.

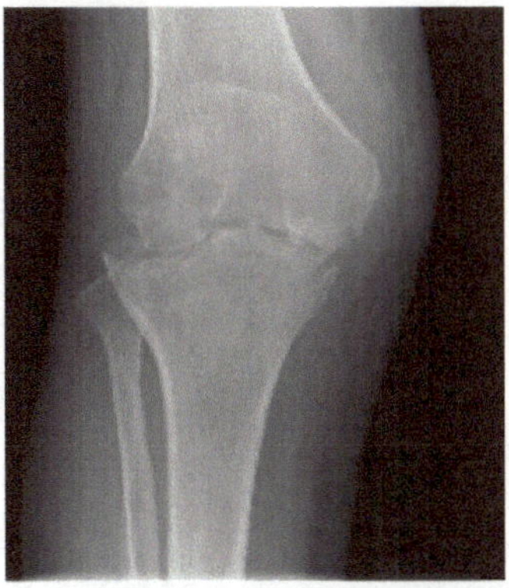

TUBERCULOSIS SPINE/ TB SPONDYLITIS

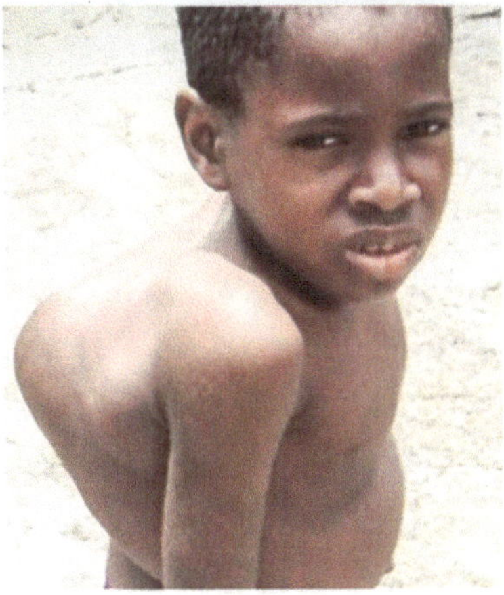

Features

- Also known as Pott's disease/ TB spondylitis.
- **Most Common** site of skeletal TB: Vertebrae.
- Skeletal TB is the third **most common** type of tuberculosis (First is TB of lungs and second is TB of lymph nodes).
- Infection reach spine because of some primary focus (lungs, lymph nodes). Bacteria reaches spine through paravertebral (Batson's plexus).
- **Most common** region involved in spinal TB: T9-L1 (Dorso-lumbar).
- **Earliest** symptom of spinal TB: Back Pain.

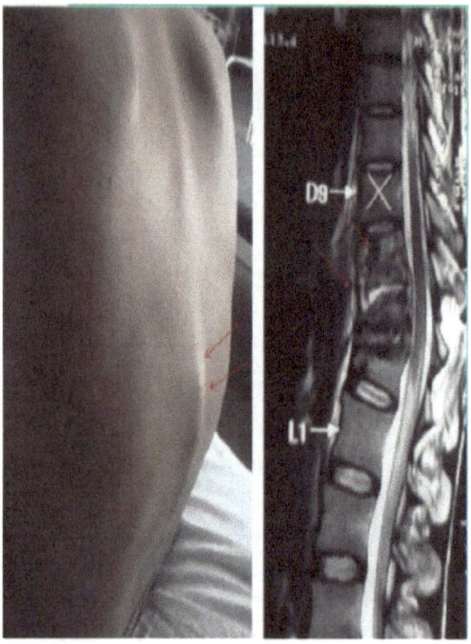

- *Other complaints:*
  - Stiffness (very early symptom).
  - Paraplegia.
  - Deformity (Gibbus/ kyphus).
  - Cold abscess.
- *Examination findings:*
  - Walks with short gait so as to avoid any jerk on the spine.
  - In dorsal spine TB, one may see a gibbus/ kyphus deformity.
  - Cold abscess may be seen as a paravertebral swelling.

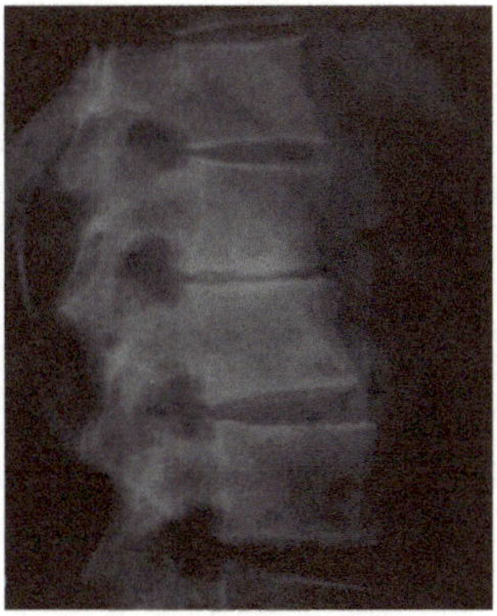

- *X-ray sign in Pott's disease/ TB spondylitis:*
    - Narrowing of disc space (This is because dying of intervertebral disc space bringing the vertebral bodies closer): Earliest radiological sign.
    - Destruction of vertebral body.
    - Cold abscess may be seen.
    - Signs of healing in late stages.

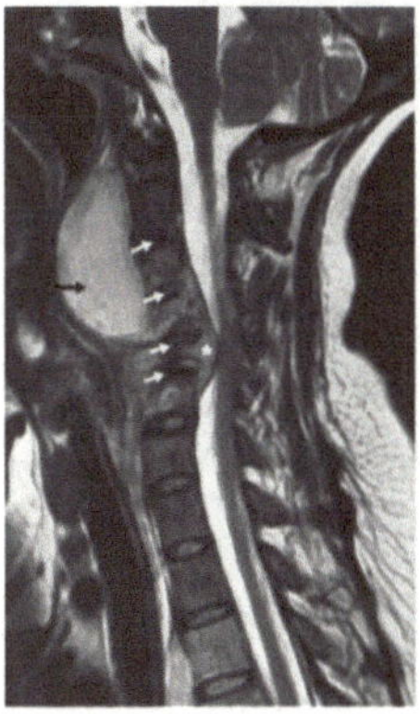

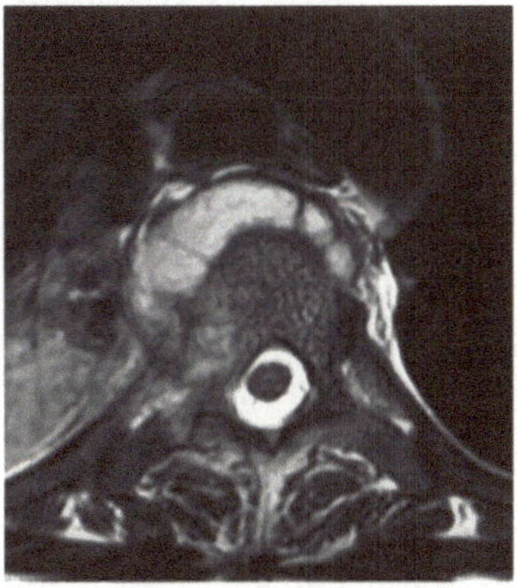

- **Most common** subtype of spinal TB is paradiscal.
    - Paradiscal means lower half of upper vertebra, intervening disc and upper half of lower vertebra. This is because typical blood supply in this fashion.
- Anterior type of vertebral TB may show erosion of anterior part of the vertebral body, just as in the case of aneurysm of aorta (**aneurysmal sign**).

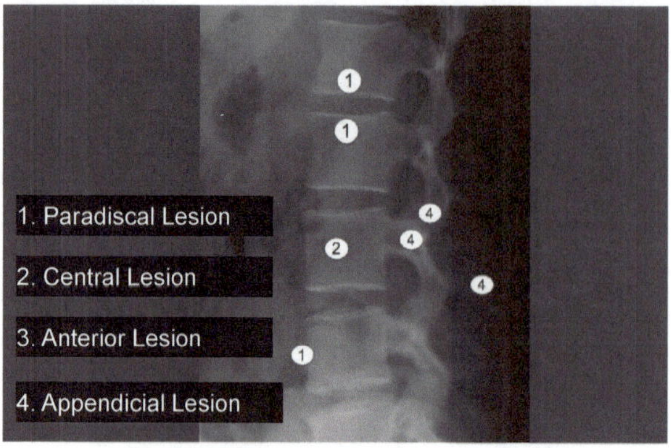

- Healing of spinal TB occurs with **bony ankylosis**.

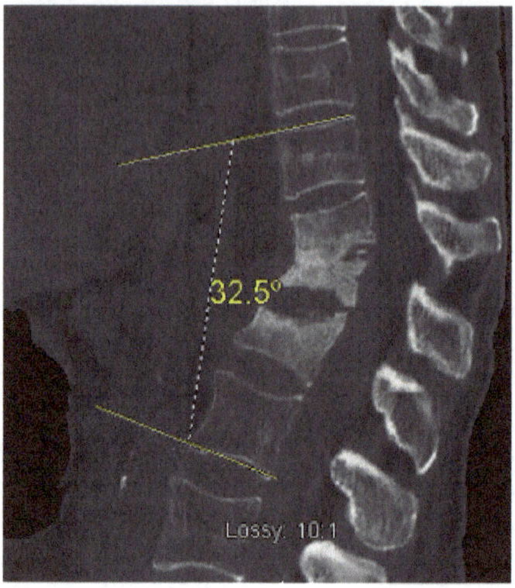

- **Pott's paraplegia**:
  - Refers to neurological complications commonly seen with thoracic spine TB where spinal cord is affected.
  - **Most commonly** seen in thoracic/dorsal spine (D1 is first dorsal vertebrae in the MRI).
  - MRI is the **investigation** of choice.
  - *Surgical procedures:*
    - Costo-transversectomy.
    - Antero-lateral decompression.

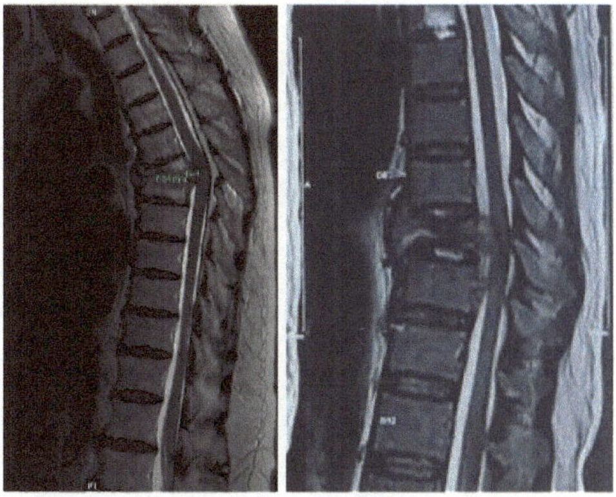

TUBERCULOSIS OF THE HIP JOINT

Features

- *Pathology:*
    - Initial lesion is in bone (unlike knee, where it is in synovium).
    - Granulation tissue (with bacilli) reaches the joint eroding the bone/ cartilage.
- **Most commonly** affects children.
- *Clinical presentation:*
    - **Night cries/ Starting pain**: Because of relaxation of muscles at night, bony surfaces rub against each other producing severe pain.
    - Pain is **referred** to knee joint because of same nerve of hip and knee joint.
    - Cold abscess in late stages may develop
- *Three stages of TB hip:*
    - Stage of apparent lengthening (synovitis): Limb is in **FABER** (**F**lexion, **AB**duction and **E**xternal **R**otation). This is the position of limb in which it can accommodate excessively produced synovial fluid, as a result of synovitis.
    - Stage of apparent shortening (stage of arthritis): Limb is in **FADIR** (**F**lexion, **A**dduction and **I**nternal **R**otation). This is because of spasm of muscles around hip due to involvement of articular cartilage. The hip flexors and adductors are more powerful so hip goes into flexion, adduction and internal rotation.

- Stage of true shortening (arthritis with bone destruction): Limb is in **FADIR.** Here the cartilage is destroyed and the head of the femur/ acetabulum is eroded. There is destruction of bone.

- Apparent lengthening means limb appears lengthened but if one measures the length of both the limbs, they are equal.
- *X-ray features:*
    - Haziness of the bone around the hip joint is the earliest sign.
    - Reduction in hip joint space.
    - Lytic lesions may be seen.
    - Irregular outlines of the articular ends of the bones.
    - **Wandering** acetabulum/ Pestle & Mortar acetabulum may be seen.

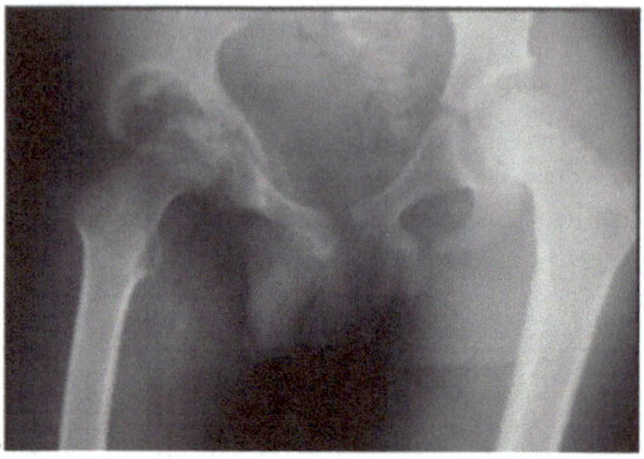

- Fixed flexion deformity at hip is judged by Thomas test.
- *Treatment:*
    - Joint debridement
    - Girdlestone arthroplasty

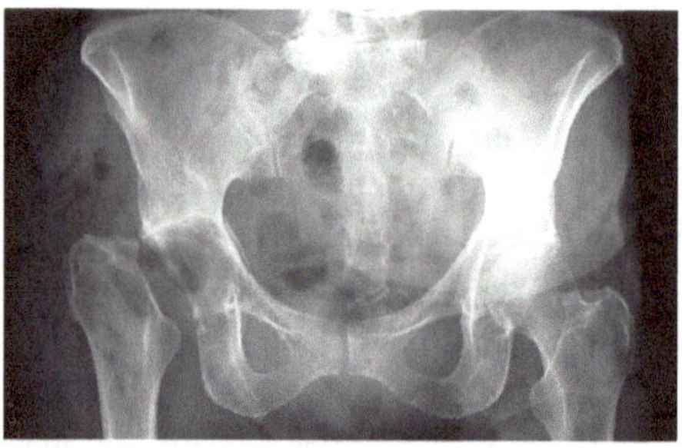

- TB hip heals by **fibrous** ankylosis.

TUBERCULOSIS OF KNEE JOINT

Features

- Begins in synovium.
- Long standing TB knee results in **triple deformity** (knee flexion, lateral rotation and posterior subluxation).

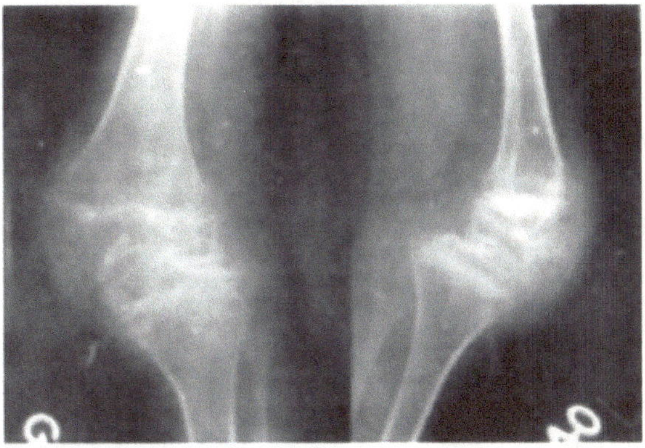

TUBERCULOUS DACTYLITIS

Features

- TB of short bones (phalanges)
- Also known as spina **ventosa**.

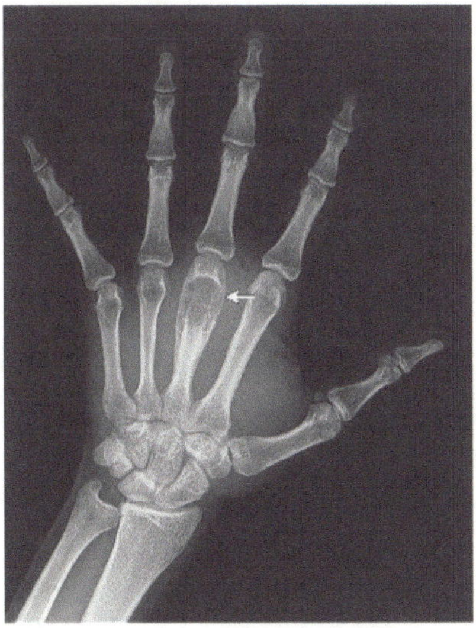

TUBERCULOSIS OF THE SHOULDER

Features

- Known as caries **sicca** as it does not produce any pus/ cold abscess.

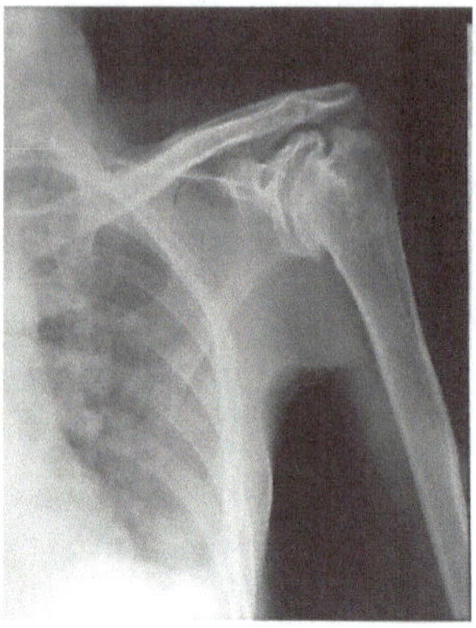

CHAPTER 4

BONY TUMOURS

LOCATION OF TUMOURS

- *Epiphyseal:*
    - Osteoclastoma
    - Chondroblastoma.
- *Metaphyseal:*
    - Osteosarcoma.
    - Osteochondroma.
    - Aneurysmal bone cyst.
- *Diaphysis:*
    - Ewing's sarcoma.
    - Osteoid osteoma.

CLASSIFICATION

Benign tumours:

Bone forming tumours	Cartilage forming tumours
Osteoma	Osteochondroma
Osteoid osteoma	Enchondroma
Osteoblastoma	
Osteoclastoma	

Malignant tumours:

Bone forming tumours	Cartilage forming tumours
Osteosarcoma	Chondrosarcoma
Ewing's sarcoma	

OSTEOID OSTEOMA

Features

- Commonest **true** benign tumour of the bone.

- Consists of a **nidus** of tangled arrays of partially mineralised osteoid trabeculae surrounded by dense sclerotic bone.
- Presenting complaint is a nagging pain, **worst** at night, and is relieved by salicylates/**Aspirin**.
- Therefore, it is also known as Aspirin tumour.
- X-ray shows a zone of sclerosis surrounding a radiolucent nidus, usually less than 1 cm in size.
- Diagnosis can be confirmed on X-ray.
- Prognosis is good.
- It is **not** a premalignant condition.

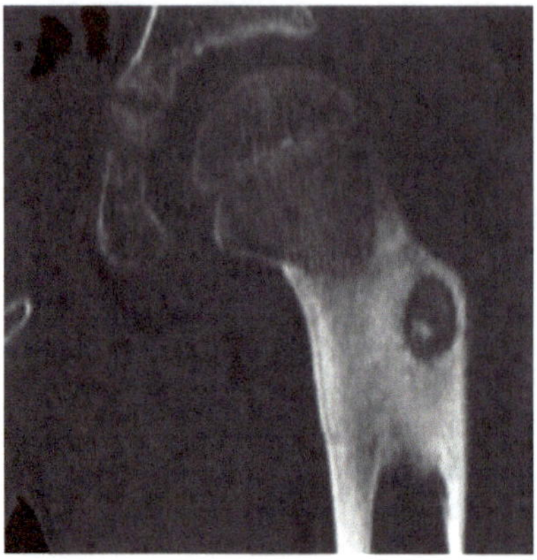

OSTEOBLASTOMA

Features

- Same as osteoid osteoma, but larger and found in vertebrae.

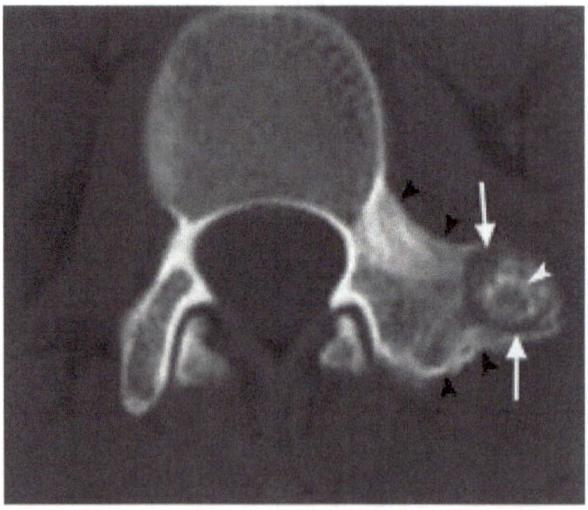

CHONDROBLASTOMA

Features

- Also known as Codman's tumour.
- Well circumscribed lesion.
- Found in epiphysis of a long bone.
- May show calcification on X-ray.

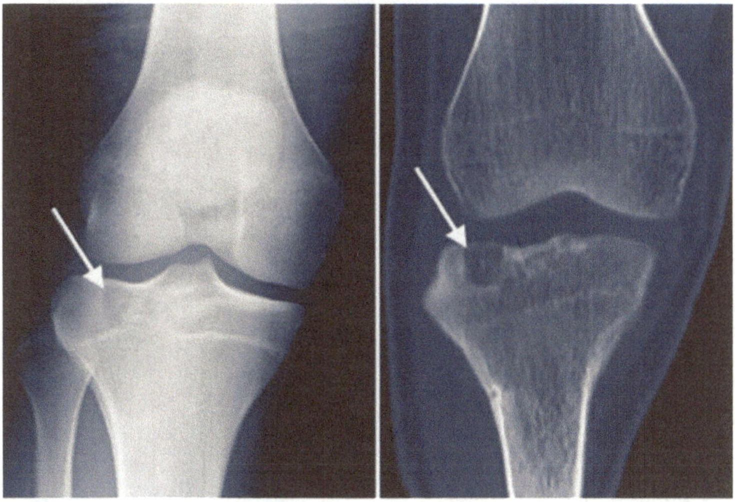

GIANT CELL TUMOUR

Features

- Commonly seen in the age group of **20-40 years**.
- Affects **epiphysis** of long bones (most commonly lower femur and upper tibia).
- *Histology:*
    - Mononuclear **spindle cells**: Tumour cells (proliferative component of the tumour).
    - Mononuclear **giant cells**: Non-tumour cells (therefore giant cell tumour is a misnomer).
- X-ray: **Soap bubble appearance**.
- Treatment: Excision of tumour with reconstruction.

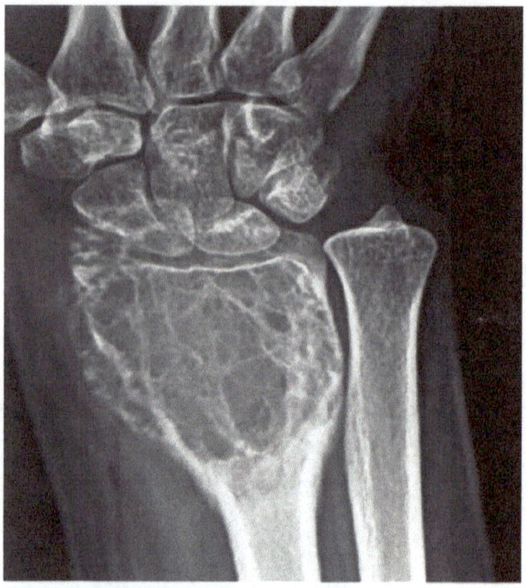

OSTEOCHONDROMA/ EXOSTOSIS

Features

- **Most common** benign tumour of bone.
- **Rarely** grows beyond the age of skeletal maturity.
- Affects male under 25 years of age.
- Originates from metaphysis of long bones, flat bones and small bones of hands and feet.
- Mature bone with cartilaginous cap seen.
- **Rare** malignant transformation to chondrosarcoma.

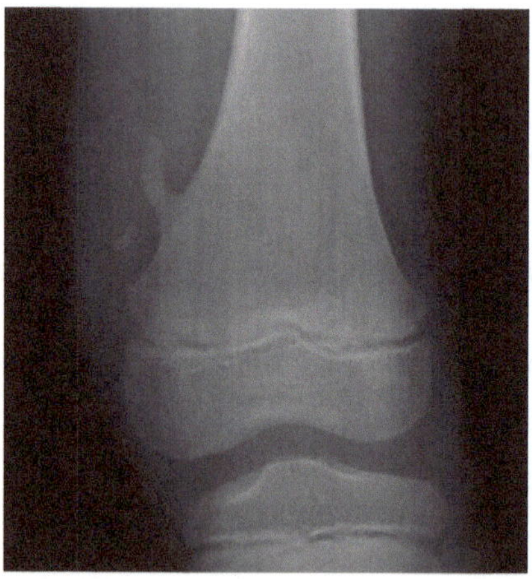

ENCHONDROMA

Features

- Arises from remnant of epiphyseal cartilage.
- Affects small bones of hands and feet.

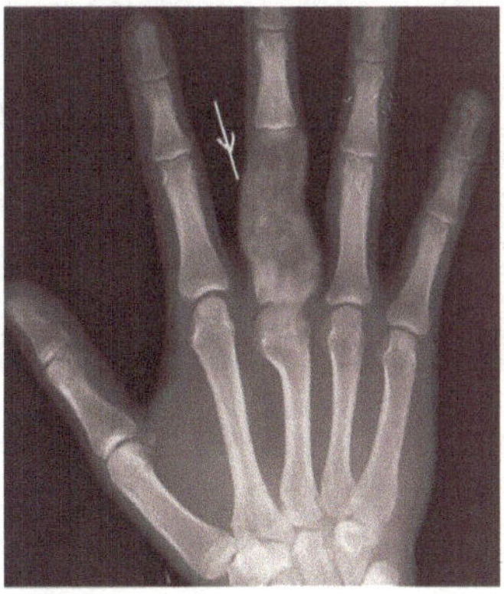

OSTEOSARCOMA

Features

- Location: Metaphysis.
- *Most common site in body (around knee joint):*
  - Lower end of femur.
  - Upper end of tibia.
- Osteosarcoma is the **second** most common primary malignant tumour of bone after multiple myeloma (**Most common** malignant tumour of bone is secondaries/ metastasis).
- Osteosarcoma is commonly seen in 15-25 years age group.
- Presents as pain and swelling of few weeks to months.
- *Predisposing conditions:*
  - Familial retinoblastoma.
  - Radiotherapy.
  - Paget's disease (adult osteosarcoma).
  - Bone infarcts.
- *X-ray appearance:*

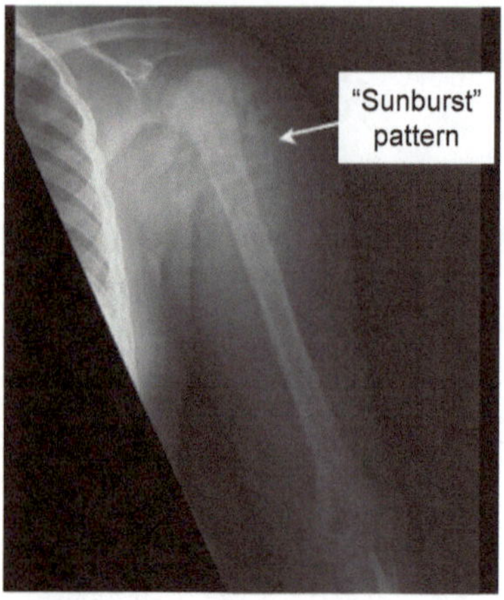

- Sunburst appearance.
- Codman's triangle.
- New bone formation.
- Lytic lesion with moth eaten appearance.

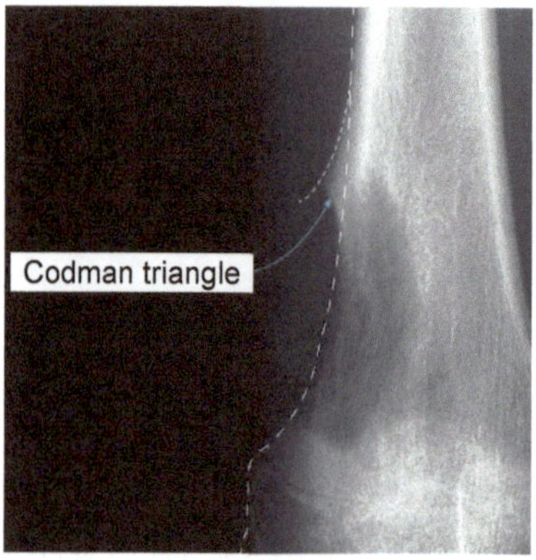

- Special feature: Secondaries in lungs.
- *Treatment:*
  - Pre-operative chemotherapy.
  - Limb salvage/sparing surgery followed by post-operative chemotherapy.
- It is extremely radio-**resistant**.
- **Poor** prognosis.

EWING SARCOMA

Features

- Anaplastic small malignant tumour.
- Location: Diaphysis.
- Age group: 2nd decade (<15 years boys).
- Pain and swelling of few weeks to months.
- X-ray appearance: **Onion** peel.
- May mimic (because of age group and region involved): Chronic osteomyelitis.
- Ewing's sarcoma affects diaphysis of long bones and flat bones.
- It is associated with 11:22 translocation.
- Extremely aggressive with early metastasis.
- It is a curable tumour as it is chemo-sensitive.

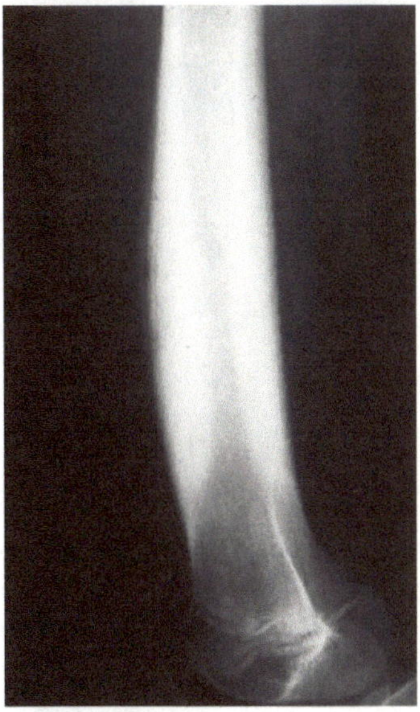

CHONDROSARCOMA

Features

- Affects men; 30-60 years.
- Affects flat bones and long bones.

- May be primary; or arise from osteochondroma.
- Presents with pain and swelling.
- *X-ray appearances:*
  - Expansile glistening mass with medullary cavity.
  - Mottled calcification within tumour.

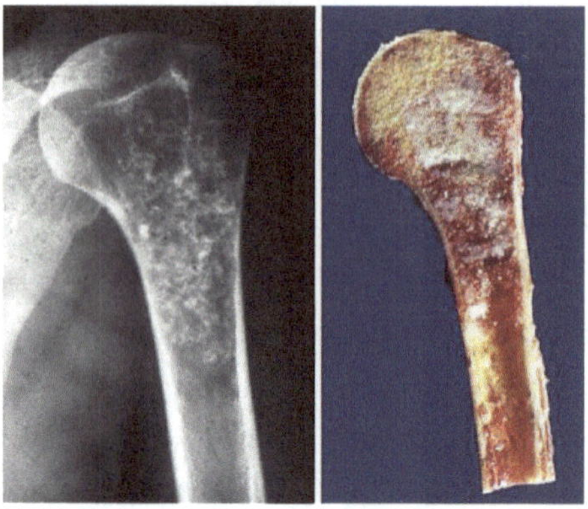

SIMPLE/ UNICAMERAL BONE CYST

Features

- Affects <20 years.
- Upper humerus is affected.
- Metaphysis.
- *X-ray appearances:*
  - Radiolucent lesions in contact with growth plate.
  - Maximum width less than width of growth plate.
  - Fallen fragment sign.

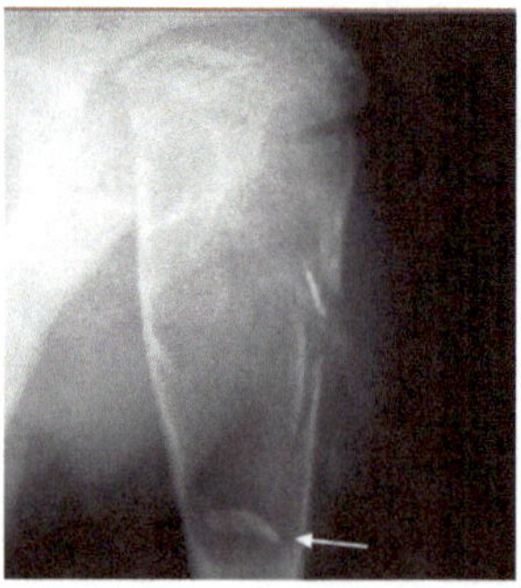

ANEURYSMAL BONE CYST

Features

- Affects 10-40 years.
- Tibia.
- Metaphysis.
- *X-ray appearances:*
  - Expansile (blood filled) lesion ballooning the bone.
  - Cyst may extend to soft tissues, simulating malignant tumour.

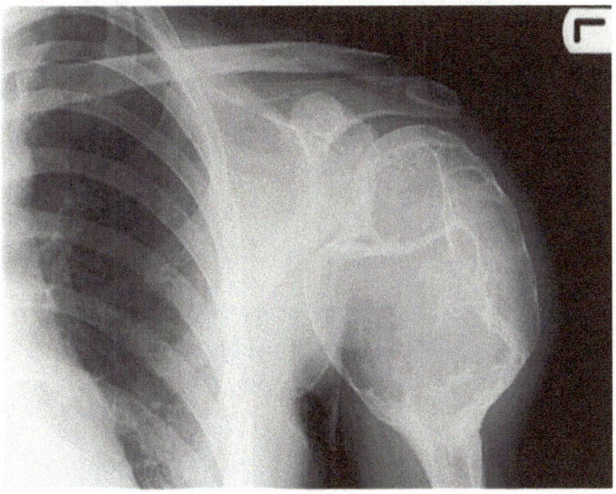

MULTIPLE MYELOMA/MM

Features

- **Most common** primary malignant bony neoplasm of the elderly aged more than 40-50 years. (Remember **Most common** malignant bony neoplasm are secondaries).
- **Bence** Jones proteins (IgG light chains) on urine electrophoresis.
- Russel bodies.
- Serum protein electrophoresis shows **M** spike (monoclonal immunoglobulin spike).
- Beta-2 microglobulin is an important prognostic indicator.
- Rouleaux formation of RBCs on peripheral smear.
- Multiple myeloma is a monoclonal **plasma cell** cancer that arises within the bone marrow (most specific test is bone marrow biopsy) and produces large amount of IgG or IgA.

- Patient presents with back pain and hypercalcemic manifestations like renal stones, renal failure etc.
- Multiple myeloma may lead to primary amyloidosis.
- **Calcium** levels: Raised.
- X-ray appearance: Geographic/**punched** out osteolytic lesion.
- Managed by Melphalan, steroids and thalidomide.

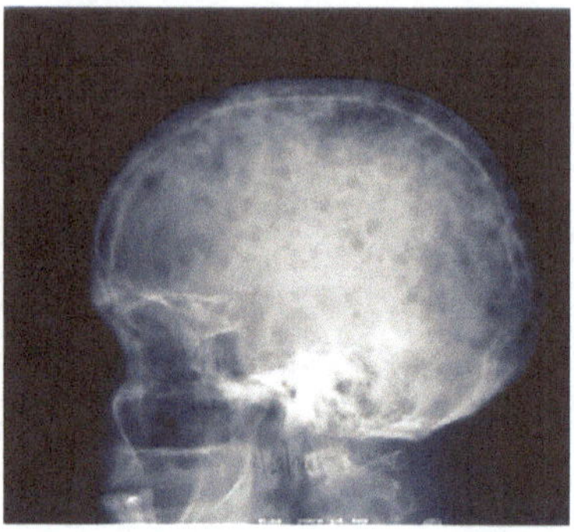

PAGET'S DISEASE/ OSTEITIS DEFORMANS

Features

- *Commonly involved bones:*
  - Pelvis (**Most common**).
  - Tibia.
  - Skull.
- In Paget's disease, there is abnormal bony architecture because of high osteoclastic and osteoblastic activity.
- Hearing loss is common due to narrowing of auditory foramen.
- *X-ray appearances:*
  - Mosaic bone pattern/ Cotton-wool areas of sclerotic bone are seen.
  - Chalk-stick fractures in long bones.
- All laboratory values are **normal** (calcium, phosphorous and parathormone) **EXCEPT** alkaline phosphatase which is raised.
- *Complications:*
  - Sarcomatous change (**osteosarcoma** or fibrosarcoma).
  - Pathological fractures.

  - Calcific aortic stenosis.
  - Hyperuricemia and urinary stones.
- *Managed by:*
  - Bisphosphates (Alendronate, risedronate etc.) inhibits osteoclast induced bone resorption.

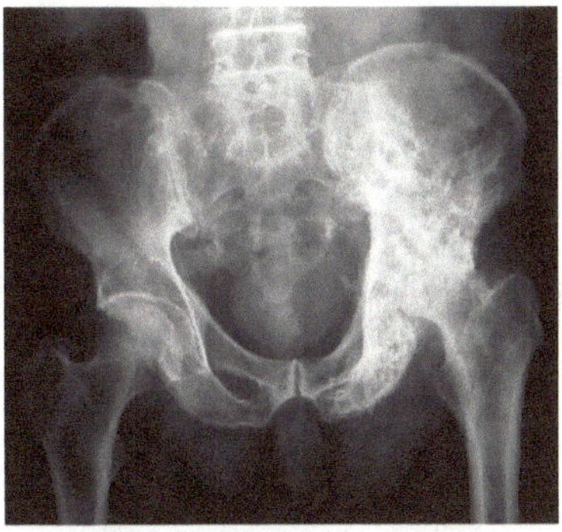

FIBROUS CORTICAL DEFECT

Features

- Also known as non-ossifying fibroma.
- Incidental finding.
- Seen in metaphyseal region of long bones.
- *X-ray appearance:*
  - Well-defined lobulated lesion.
  - Eccentrically located in the metaphysis.

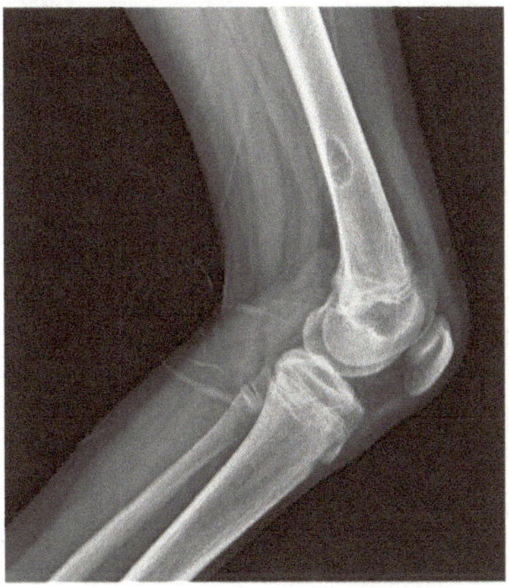

FIBROUS DYSPLASIA

Features

- Affects 20-30 years.
- Mainly affects proximal femur.
- Location: Metaphysis.
- Curettage and bone graft is done.
- *X-ray appearances:*
    - **Shepherd's** crook deformity (proximal femur).
    - Multiloculated ground glass appearance.
    - Trabeculations.

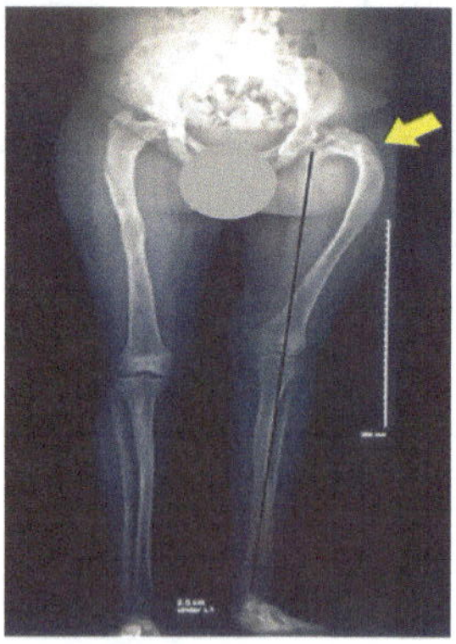

CHONDROMYXOID FIBROMA

Features

- Affects 10-30 years old.
- Most commonly seen in proximal tibia.
- Calcification is usually **absent**.

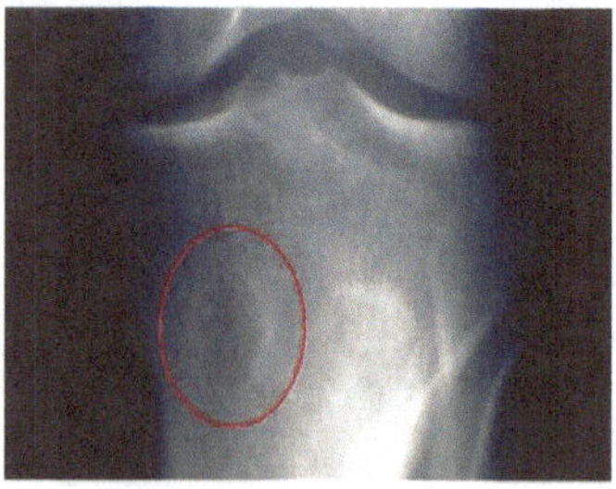

HEMANGIOMA OF BONE

Features

- Benign lesion
- *CT scan:*
    - Transverse section: Polka dot pattern.
    - Lateral view: Jailhouse/ Corduroy appearance/ Linear striations.

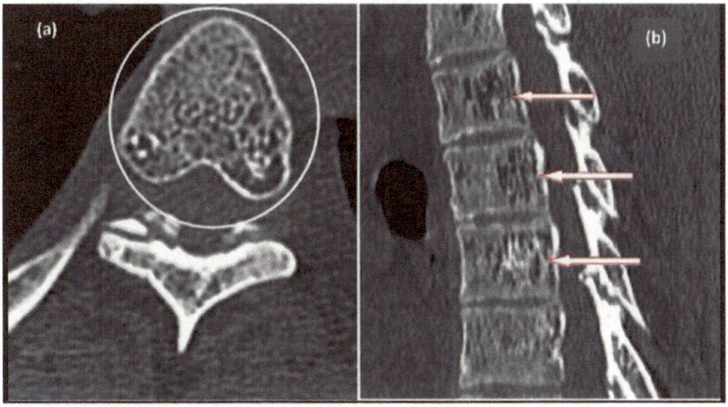

METASTATIS TO BONES

Features

- *Most common site of primary carcinomas:*
    - Males: Carcinoma prostate.
    - Females: Carcinoma breast.
- Most commonly site of bony metastasis is dorsal/ thoracic vertebrae.
- *Types:*
    - Osteolytic:
        - Carcinoma kidney.
        - Carcinoma thyroid.
    - Osteoblastic:
        - Carcinoma prostate.

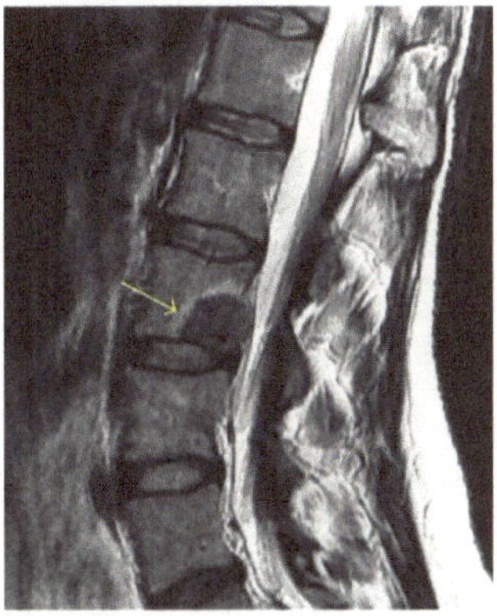

CHAPTER 5

PERIPHERAL NERVE INJURIES

BRACHIAL PLEXUS

Parts:

- **R**oots.
- **T**runks.
- **D**ivision.
- **C**ords.

Location:

- Roots and trunks in neck.
- Divisions behind the clavicle.
- Cords in axilla.

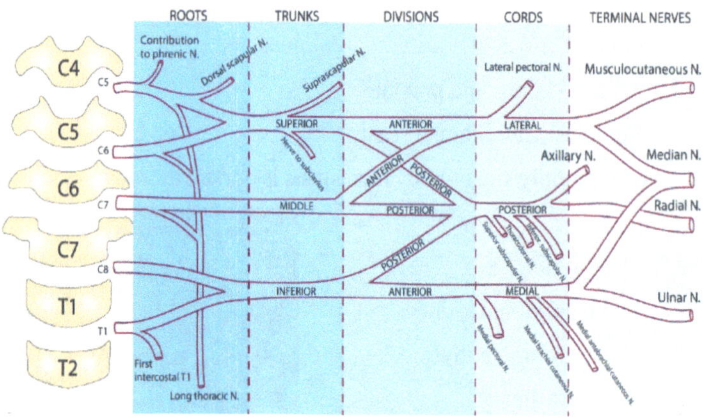

Injuries:

- Upper trunk injury: Policeman's tip hand.
- Lower trunk injury: Klumpke's palsy.
- Long thoracic nerve injury: Winging of scapula.

Deformities following nerve injuries:

- Ape hand: Median nerve injury.
- Partial clawing: Ulnar nerve injury.
- Complete clawing: Both ulnar and median nerve injury.
- Wrist drop: Radial nerve injury.

Erb's palsy:

- Involves upper trunk of brachial plexus.
- *Nerves and Muscles paralyzed:*
    - Suprascapular nerve (Supraspinatus and Infraspinatus)
    - Axillary nerve (Deltoid and Teres minor).
    - Musculocutaneous nerve (Biceps brachii, coracobrachialis and brachioradialis).
    - Nerve to subclavius (Subclavius muscle).
- *Waiters tip deformity/ Policeman tip deformity:*
    - Loss of abduction of arm (Deltoid and supraspinatus).
    - Loss of lateral rotation of arm (Teres minor and infraspinatus).
    - Loss of flexion of elbow (Biceps brachii, coracobrachialis and brachioradialis).

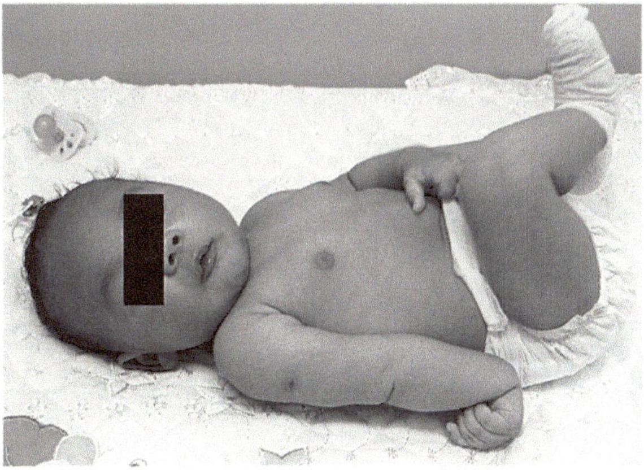

Klumpke's paralysis:

- Injury to lower trunk of brachial plexus (C8, T1).
- Results in clawing of hand and Horner's syndrome.

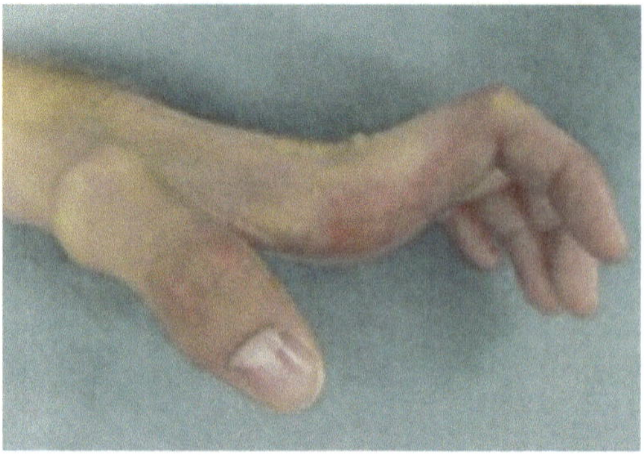

AXILLARY NERVE

Features

- *Injured in:*
  - Anterior dislocation of shoulder.
  - Fracture surgical neck of humerus.
  - Faulty intramuscular injections in deltoid.
- Regiment badge sign: Anaesthesia on the lateral part of arm.
- Weakness of shoulder abduction because of paralysis of deltoid.

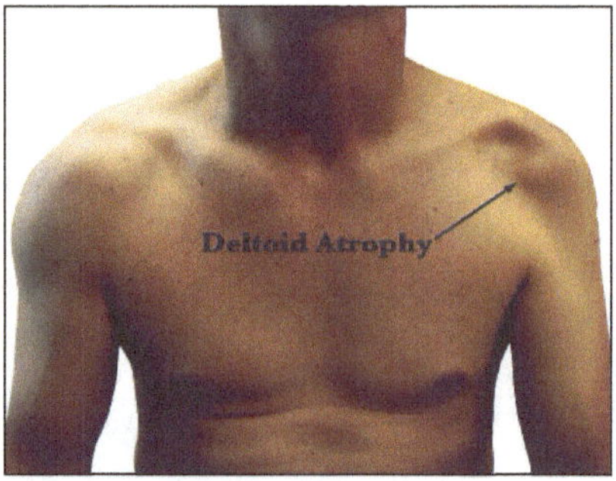

MUSCULOCUTANEOUS NERVE

Muscles Supplied (Mnemonic: BBC):

- Biceps brachii.
- Brachialis.
- Coracobrachialis.

Injury of results in:

- Loss of flexion of elbow
- Supination of forearm
- Sensory loss on the lateral aspect of forearm

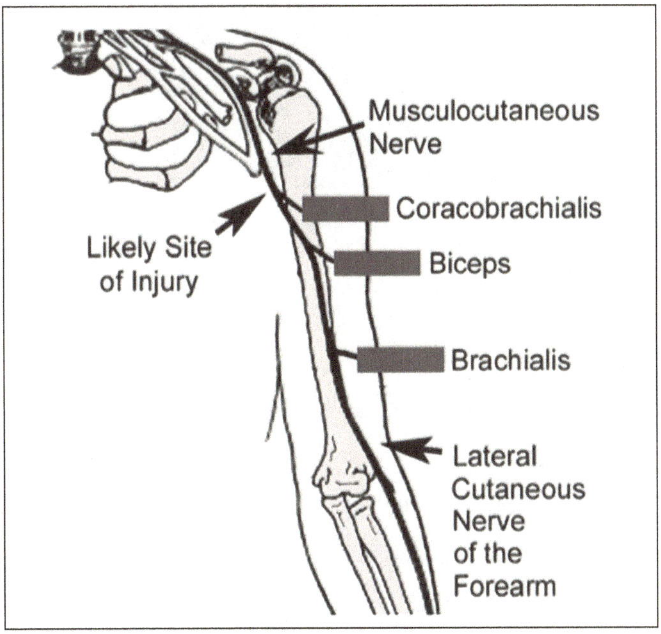

RADIAL NERVE

Muscles Supplied by radial nerve:

- Triceps.
- Extensors of metacarpo-phalangeal joint (Extensor compartment of arm and forearm).
- Anconeus.

Injury of radial nerve in axillary part:

- Loss of elbow extension
- Wrist drop
- Finger drop
- Loss of cutaneous sensations

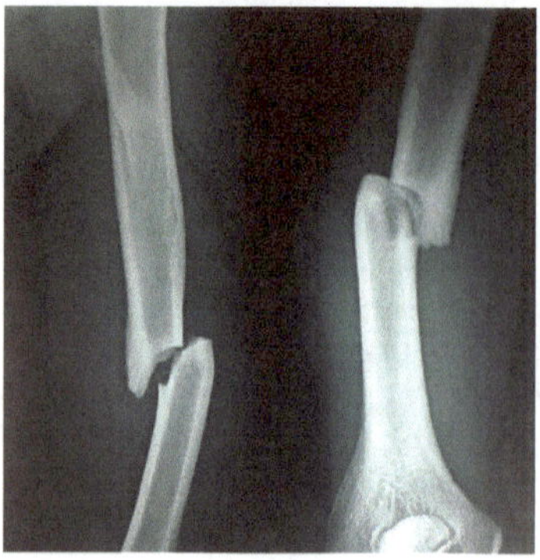

Injury of radial nerve in fracture shaft of humerus:

- Wrist drop.
- Finger drop.
- Loss of cutaneous sensations.

Injury of radial nerve in forearm:

- Finger drop.
- Loss of cutaneous sensations.

Injury of radial nerve at wrist:

- Loss of cutaneous sensations.

Features:

- Saturday night palsy.
- Crutch palsy.
- Paralysis of radial nerve results in wrist drop (paralysis of extensors of wrists and fingers).

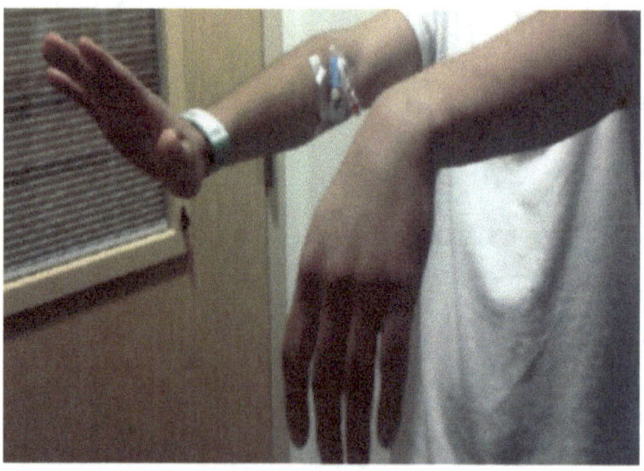

MEDIAN/ LABOURER'S NERVE

Muscle supplied by median nerve in forearm:

- All muscles of flexor compartment of forearm **except** medial half of flexor digitorum profundus.

Muscle supplied by median nerve in hand (Mnemonic: LOFA):

- 1st and 2nd **L**umbrical.
- **O**pponens pollicis.
- **F**lexor pollicis brevis.
- **A**bductor pollicis brevis.

Median nerve injury results in:

- Ape thumb deformity.
- Pointing index.
- Loss of opposition and thumb abduction.

Features:

- Wasting of thenar eminence.
- **Ape** thumb/simian deformity.
- **Pointing** index/Ochsner clasping test: Paralysis of FDP (flexor digitorum profundus) and FDS (flexor digitorum superficialis) of the index finger.
- **Pen** test: Patient is told to abduct the thumb and touch a pen placed at a distance. This checks abductor pollicis **brevis**.

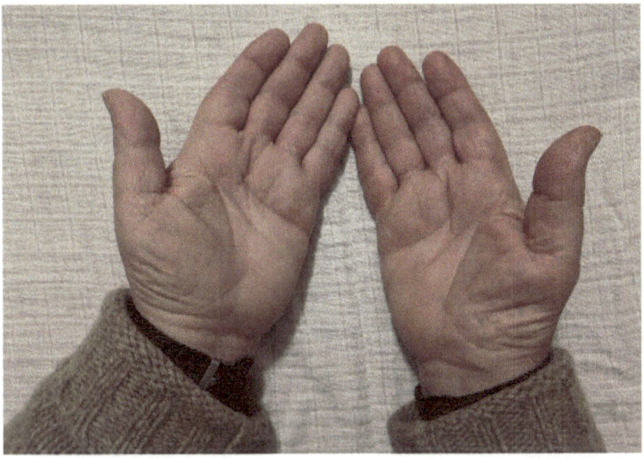

CARPAL TUNNEL SYNDROME/ CTS

Features

- CTS is because of compression of median nerve as it passes beneath the flexor retinaculum.
- *Causes of CTS (Mnemonic: CARPAL-MD)*:
  - **C**olle's fracture.
  - **A**cromegaly.
  - **R**heumatoid arthritis.
  - **P**regnancy.
  - **A**myloidosis.
  - **L**ow thyroid (hypothyroidism).
  - **M**yxedema.
  - **D**islocation of lunate bone.
- Patient presents with complaints of tingling in the lateral two and a half fingers. Later on, there may be wasting of thenar eminence and decreased sensation over lateral three and a half fingers on volar side.
- *Phalen's test:*
  - If the wrist is palmar-flexed for 1 minute, compression of median nerve will occur and this will lead to production of symptoms.
  - Straightening of wrist leads to disappearance of symptoms.
- Managed by either steroid injections or decompression surgery by dividing flexor retinaculum.

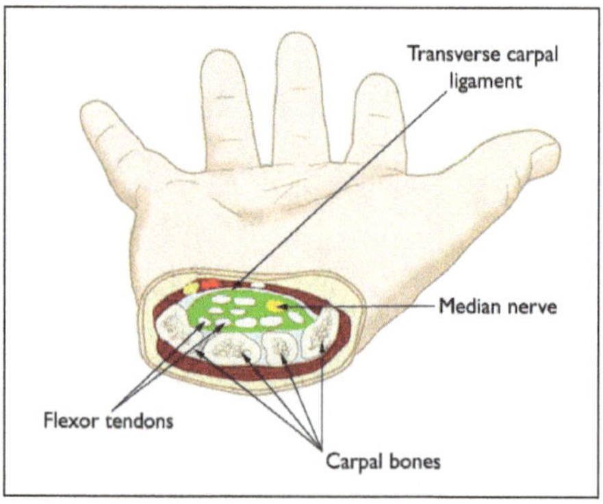

ULNAR/ MUSICIAN'S NERVE

Muscle supplied by ulnar nerve in hand:

- *All muscles except **LOFA**:*
    - 1st and 2nd **L**umbrical.
    - **O**pponens pollicis.
    - **F**lexor pollicis brevis.
    - **A**bductor pollicis brevis.

Cubital tunnel syndrome:

- Compression neuropathy of ulnar nerve.
- Ulnar nerve pierces flexor carpi ulnaris and can be compressed.

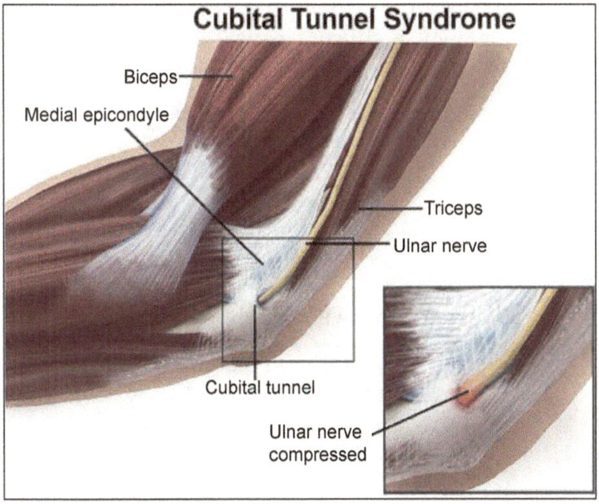

Injury of ulnar nerve results in:

- Partial clawing of hand.
- Involving 4th and 5th finger.

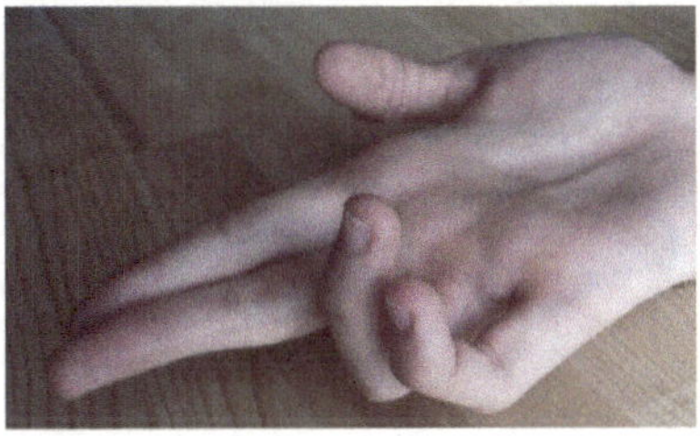

Clinical tests related to ulnar nerve:

- Book test/Froment's sign.
- Egawa test.
- Card test.

Features:

- Positive **card** test (weak palmar interossei; patient is unable to hold card between fingers).
- Ulnar **claw** hand (partial claw hand if only ulnar nerve is injured; total clawing is seen if both the ulnar and median nerves are injured).
- Egawa test (weak dorsal interossei; patient is unable to abduct middle finger/fingers against resistance).
- *Book test/Froment's sign:* Ulnar nerve palsy leads to paralysis of adductor pollicis and hence patient uses flexor pollicis longus (supplied by median nerve) to hold the book kept in first webspace.

COMMON PERONEAL NERVE INJURY

Features

- Commonly injured in fracture of neck of fibula.
- Muscles of anterior and lateral compartment of the leg are paralyzed.
- Patient clinically presents with foot drop.

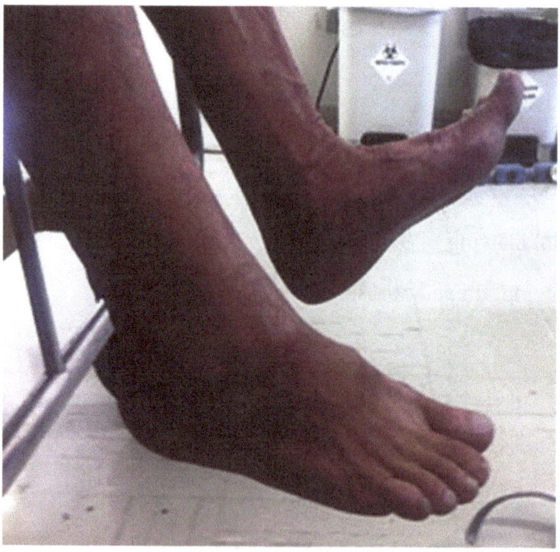

TARSAL TUNNEL SYNDROME

Features

- Compression of posterior tibial nerve behind the flexor retinaculum.
- Patient presents with burning sensation and paresthesia over the plantar surface of the foot.

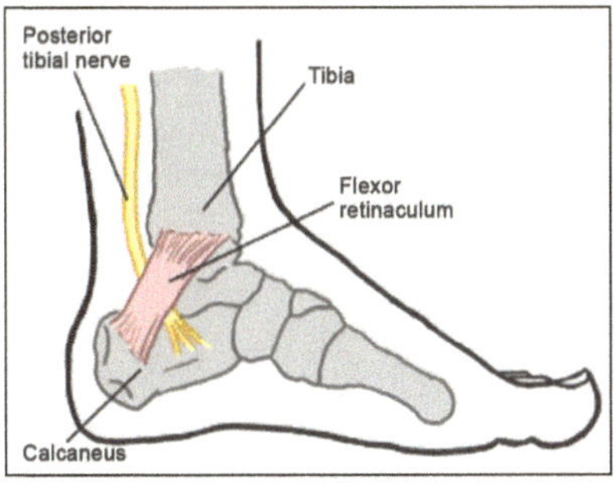

THORACIC OUTLET SYNDROME

Features

- Associated with cervical rib syndrome.
- Patient presents with features of compression of C8 ad T1 or vascular symptoms (Raynaud's phenomenon).
- Adson's test is done.

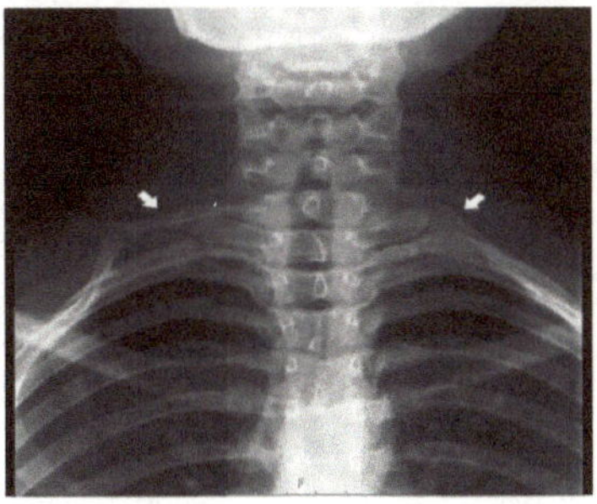

NEURAPRAXIA

Features

- Complete recovery is possible.
- Anatomical continuity normal.
- Physiological cessation of activity.

Table: Peripheral nerve injury classification and treatment

Seddon classification	Sunderland classification	Description	Myclin	Axon	Endoneurium	Perineurium	Epineurium	Treatment
Neurapraxia	I	Conduction block	Injured	Intact	Intact	Intact	Intact	Nonsurgical
Axonotmesis	II	Axon discontinuity	Injured	Injured	Intact	Intact	Intact	Nonsurgical
	III	Scarring of endoneurium	Injured	Injured	Injured	Intact	Intact	Often nonsurgical
	IV	Neuromain continuity	Injured	Injured	Injured	Injured	Intact	Surgical
Neurotmesis	V	Rupture of the nerve	Injured	Injured	Injured	Injured	Injured	Surgical

CONDITION/ INJURIES AND NERVES INVOLVED

Conditions/ Injuries and Nerves involved

- Meralgia paresthetica involves: Lateral cutaneous nerve of thigh.
- Winging of scapula involves: Long thoracic nerve of Bell.
- Foot drop: Common peroneal nerve (Related to neck of fibula).
- Supracondylar fracture (#) of humerus: Median nerve (Anterior interosseous nerve).
- Tarsal tunnel syndrome: Posterior tibial nerve entrapment.

CHAPTER 6

METABOLIC DISORDERS OF BONE

RICKETS

Features

- Defective mineralization of osteoid/ bones and cartilage because of relative or absolute deficiency of vitamin-D.
- Increased unclarified osteoid in the immature skeletal framework
- Presents by 3 – 7 months of age.
- Craniotabes (flattening of the occiput and accumulation of osteoid in the frontal and parietal regions).
- Wide open fontanelle.
- Rachitic rosary (Cupping of anterior ends of ribs and enlargement of costochondral junction).
- Bowing of legs (genu varum or wind-swept deformity).
- Triradiate pelvis.
- Harrison's sulcus (retraction of lower part of chest wall because of soft ribs).
- *X-ray:*
  - Widening and thickening of epiphysis/growth plate.
  - Cupping, splaying and fraying of metaphysis is the earliest change seen at lower ends of radius and ulna.
- Administration of vitamin D 6 lakhs unit as a single dose induces rapid healing.

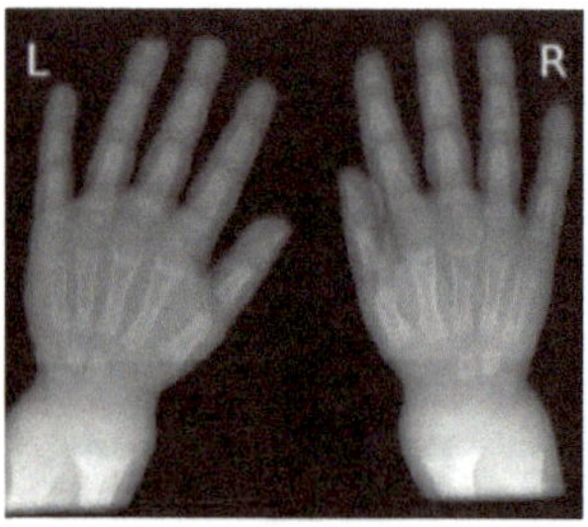

OSTEOMALACIA

Features

- Deficiency of vitamin D in adults
- Patient usually presents with low back and thigh pain
- *X-ray appearance:*
    - Looser's zone/ pseudo-fractures.
    - Triradiate pelvis.
    - Protrusio acetabuli.

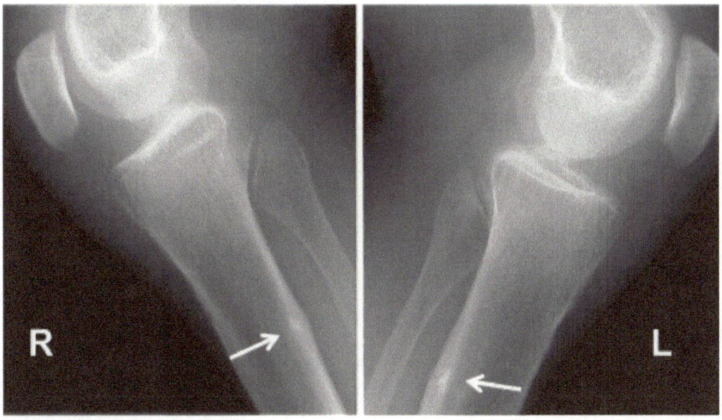

OSTEOPOROSIS

Features

- **Commonest** metabolic disease.
- Characterized by a diffuse **reduction** in the bone density due to decrease in the bone mass.
- It occurs when the rate of bone resorption exceeds the rate of bone formation.
- *X-rays:*
    - **Loss** of vertical height of a vertebra due to collapse.
    - **Cod fish** appearance.
    - **Ground glass** appearance of the bones.
- *Densitometry:*
    - Method to quantify osteoporosis.

- Absorption of photons by the bone calcium is measured.
- 2 types:
  - USG based.
  - X-ray based:
    - DEXA is X-ray based bone densitometry and is the **gold standard** in the quantification of bone mass.

- *Biochemistry:*
  - Serum Calcium, phosphates and alkaline phosphatase: All **normal.**
- *Treatment:*
  - Vitamin D and calcium.
  - Calcitonin (as parenteral or **nasal spray**).
  - **Raloxifene** (SERM/ selective estrogen receptor modulator) minimizes the risk of vertebral fractures but can cause thromboembolism or hot flushes.
  - **Alendronate** are used in once-a-day dose, empty stomach, but esophagitis is a troublesome complication.
  - **Teripartide** (Parathormone analogue) acts by stimulating the production of new collagenous bone matrix that must be mineralized and therefore sufficient **supplementation** of calcium and vitamin D3 is a must.
  - **Denosumab** is a monoclonal antibody that acts by inhibiting the proliferation and maturation of pre-osteoclasts into mature osteoclast bone resorbing cells. It acts by binding to the osteoclast receptor activator of nuclear factor kappa-B ligand (RANKL).
  - Glucocorticoids are **contraindicated**.

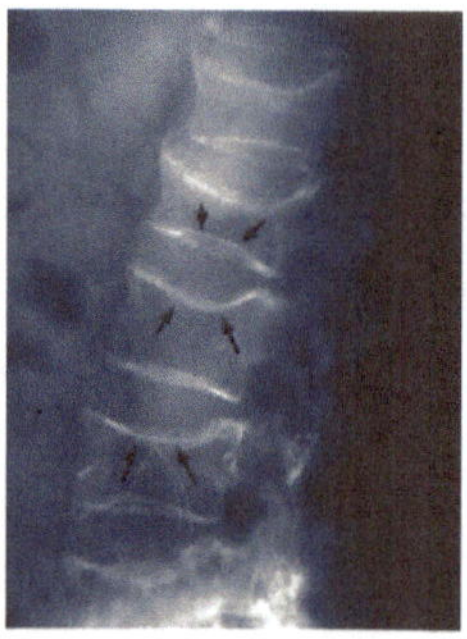

OSTEOPETROSIS

Features

- Also known as Marble bone disease.
- There is functional deficiency of osteoclast so no bony resorption takes place.
- Autosomal dominant pattern.
- X-ray shows raised radio-opacity of bones and intramedullary canal is filled with bone.

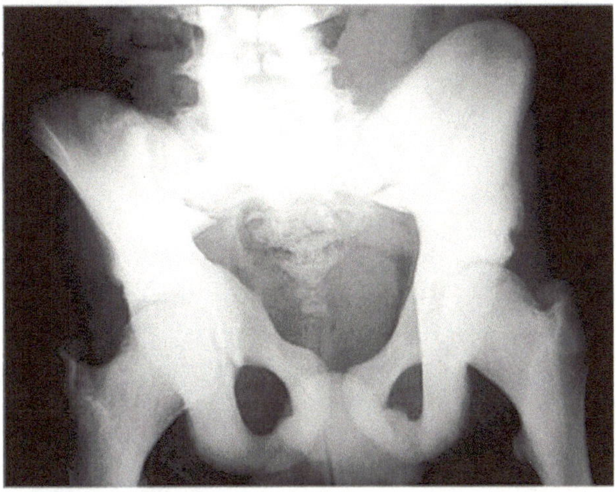

HYPERPARATHYROIDISM

Features

- MC cause is parathyroid adenoma.
- *Clinical presentation:*
    - Weak bones.
    - Abdominal groans (dyspepsia).
    - Psychic moans.
    - Renal stones.
- *X-ray appearance:*
    - Subperiosteal resorption of terminal tufts of phalanges.
    - Brown tumour.

	Calcium	Phosphate	Alkaline Phosphatase (ALP)	Parathyroid Hormone (PTH)
Osteogenesis Imperfecta	Normal	Normal	Normal	Normal
Osteoporosis	Normal	Normal	Normal	Normal
Osteomalacia	↓	↓	↑	↑
Paget's disease of bone	Normal	Normal	↑ (Isolated raised ALP)	Normal
Primary hyperparathyroidism	↑	↓	↑	↑
Secondary hyperparathyroidism	↓	↑	↑	↑
Tertiary hyperparathyroidism	↑	↑	↑	↑
Hypoparathyroidism	↑	↑	↑	↓

SCRUVY

Features

- Because of deficiency of vitamin C.
- Gums may be spongy and bleeding.
- Subperiosteal hemorrhages causes severe pain near large joints, resulting in pseudo-paralysis/frog like posture.

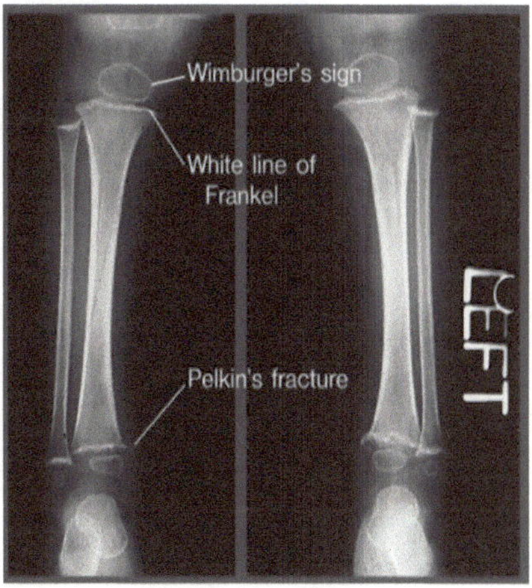

- *X-ray appearance:*
    - Osteopenia.
    - Frankel's line.
    - Wimberger's sign.
    - Pelkan spur.
    - Trummerfeld zone.

FLUOROSIS

Features

- High levels of fluorine in water result fluorosis.
- Patient presented with dental caries.
- X-ray shows calcification of interosseous membrane in forearm.

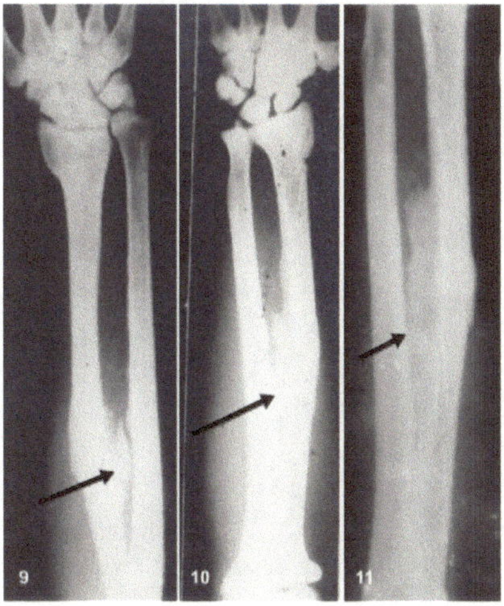

ACHONDROPLASIA

Features

- **Most common** cause of disproportionate dwarfism.
- Autosomal dominant.
- X-ray pelvis shows champagne glass pelvis.

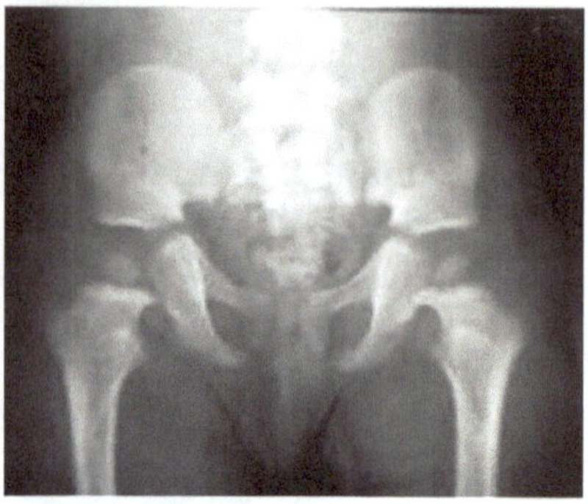

OSTEOGENESIS IMPERFECTA

Features

- Also known as Brittle bone disease.
- Autosomal dominant inheritance.
- There are repeated chances of fracture.
- Femur is the **commonest** bone to fracture.
- Blue sclera may be seen.

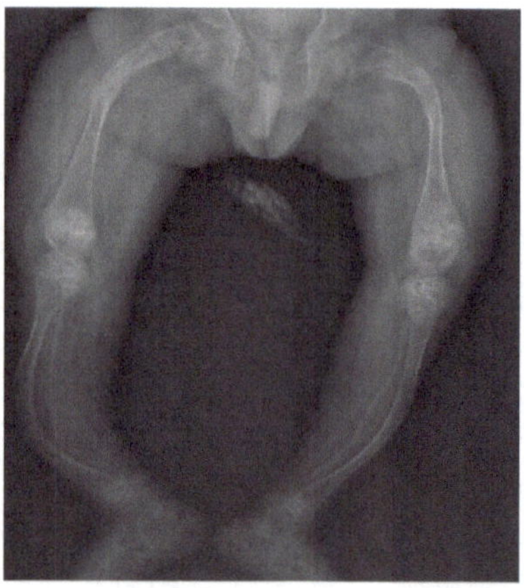

CHAPTER 7

JOINT DISORDERS

RHEUMATOID ARTHRITIS/ RA

Features

- RA is a disease of: **Synovium**/synovial membrane.
- There is hypertrophy of synovium with formation of granulation tissue over cartilage (pannus).
- RA is an autoimmune condition with inflammation of synovium/ joint.
- Associated with **HLA**-DR4.
- There is **symmetrical** hypertrophy of small joints of hands (MCP and PIP, but never DIP).
- Patients comes with the complaints of **morning** stiffness which gets better with exercise/movements.
- Ulnar deviation of fingers may occur.
- Most **dangerous** complication is atlanto-axial subluxation.
- Managed by NSAIDS, steroids, DMARDS/disease modifying anti-rheumatoid drugs like methotrexate, chloroquine, sulfasalazine, gold salts etc.
- **Mostly** affects: Females (three times).
- *Joints characteristically involved in RA:*
    - MCP (metacarpophalangeal).
    - PIP (proximal interphalangeal).
- *Boutonniere deformity:*
    - Flexion contracture of the PIP.
    - Extension of DIP (distal interphalangeal).
- *Swan neck deformity:*
    - Opposite of Boutonniere deformity i.e.

  - Extended PIP and
  - Flexed DIP
- Extra-articular manifestations are seen in: Individuals with high titres of RA Factor (IgM autoantibodies to the Fc component of IgG).

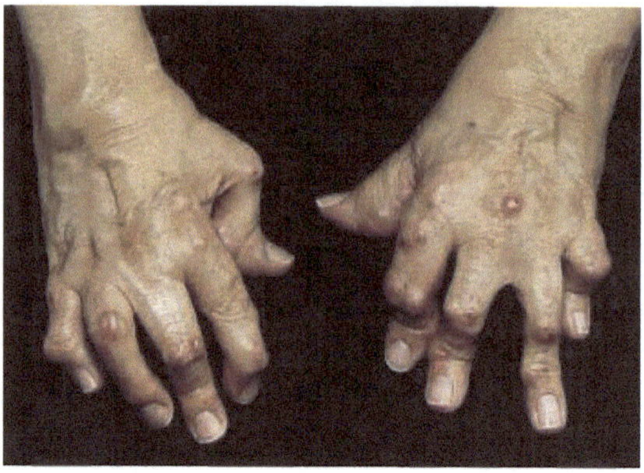

OSTEOARTHRITIS

Features

- *Usually OA involves:*
  - Hip (in western world),
  - **Knee** (in Indian setup)
- Does **not** affect MCP joint (which is most common joint affected in rheumatoid arthritis).
- *Interphalangeal joints & nodes:*
  - DIP: Heberdens node;
  - PIP: Bouchard nodes
- *X-ray shows:*
  - Osteophyte formation/ bony spur/growth of surrounding bone.
  - Narrowing of joint space (because of degeneration of cartilage and the bony surfaces they come closer).
  - Fibrillation and degeneration of cartilage.
  - Subchondral sclerosis.

- *Types:*
    - Primary:
        - **Most common** type
        - No known cause
    - Secondary:
        - Occurs because of mismanaged articular fractures, inflammatory arthropathy etc.
- *Clinical feature:*
    - **Asymmetric** arthritis (recall symmetric arthritis of rheumatoid arthritis).
    - Joint crepitus.
    - Pain along joint line (initially with activity and but later on even at rest).
- *Management:*
    - NSAIDs.
    - Intra-articular steroid injections.
    - For rest pain, arthroplasty (joint replacement).

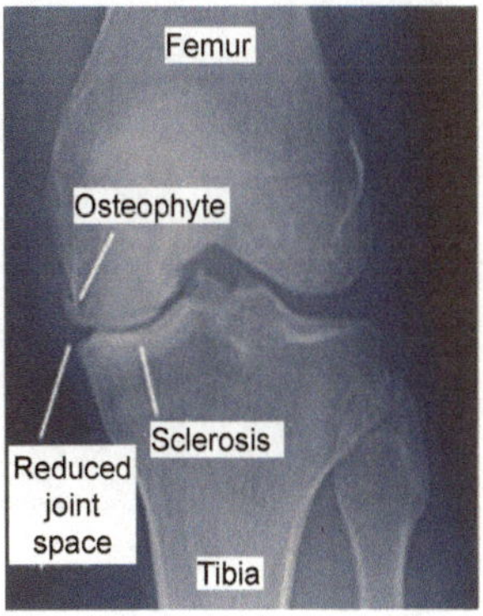

ANKYLOSING SPONDYLITIS

Features

- Also known as Marie Strumpell disease/Bechterew's disease.
- Associated HLA: **HLA B27**.
- **Enthesitis** (point of attachment of tendons/cartilage to bone is painful).

- Enthesopathy (especially around pelvis and heel).
- Affects **young** adults.
- Presents with **Back-pain** and **stiffness**, which comes with rest and tend to go away with movement.
- There is limitation of flexion and extension of lumbar spine.
- Extra-articular manifestations include acute **anterior uveitis** (most common and occurs in about one-third cases of AS), inflammatory bowel disease etc.
- To measure lumbar spine flexion, Schober test is done.
- *X-ray shows:*
    - **Bamboo spine**.
    - **Earliest** radiological change is haziness of sacro-iliac spine (**sacro-ilitis**).
    - Squaring of vertebra.
- **No** specific therapy is available.

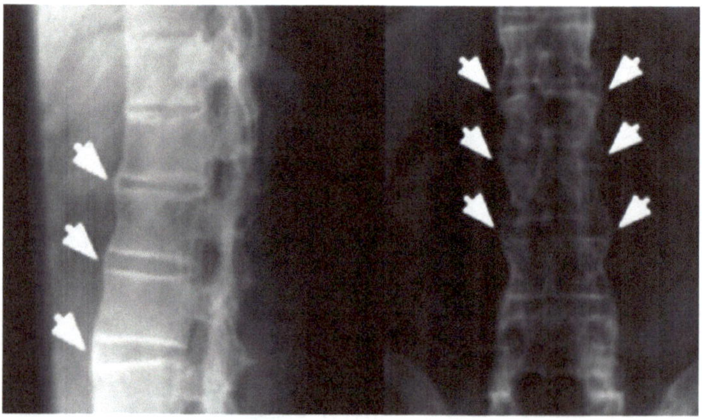

PSORIATIC ARTHRITIS

Features

- Arthritis of distal interphalangeal joint.
- Arthritis mutilans.
- Shortening of digits (telescoping).
- *X-ray:* Pencil cup deformity.

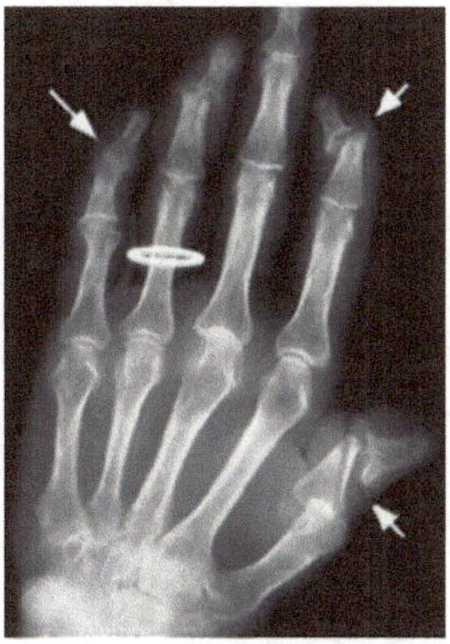

GOUT

Features

- Deposition of monosodium urate monohydrate crystals in joints.
- Associated with hyperuricemia.
- **Most common** site is metatarsophalangeal joint of big toe.
- The skin is shiny, swollen with raised temperature and very tender.
- Synovial fluid examination: Demonstrates negatively birefringent urate crystals (under polarized light), which are needle or rod shaped.
- *Management:*
  - Acute attack: NSAIDs, colchicine.
  - Chronic cases: Allopurinol (Inhibitor of xanthine oxidase).

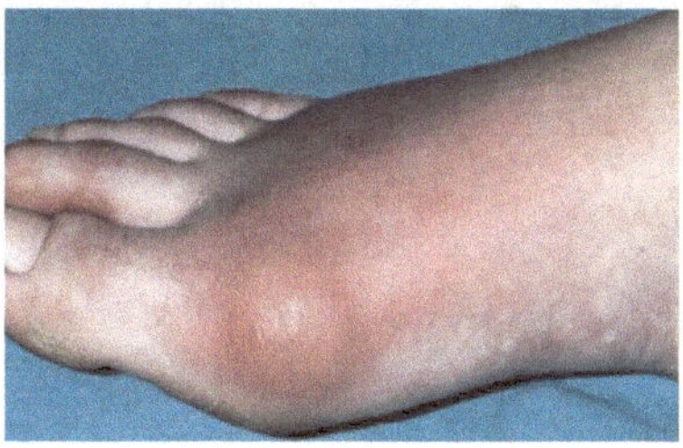

PSEUDO-GOUT

Features

- Deposition of calcium pyrophosphate/CPPD crystal.
- Affects larger joints (knee).

- Commonly seen in hypothyroidism.
- Synovial fluid examination: Demonstrates positive birefringent CPPD crystals (under polarized light), which are rhomboid shaped.

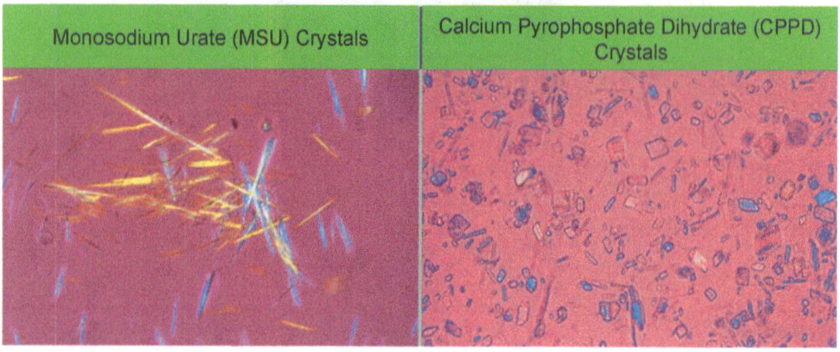

NEUROPATHIC JOINT DISEASE

Features

- Also known as Charcot's joint.
- Commonly seen in diabetes mellitus.
- Joint is markedly swollen and deformed but is non-tender.

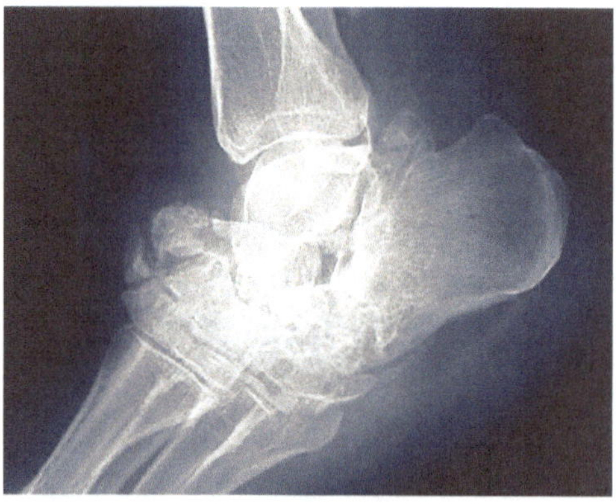

HEMOPHILIC ARTHROPATHY

Features

- Hemophilia is due to deficiency of factor VIII (hemophilia-A/Classical) or IX (hemophilia-B/Christmas disease).
- X-linked recessive disorder.
- Bleeding commonly occurs in knee joint.

- Intramuscular bleeding can occur.
- *Management:*
    - Replacement of deficient factor.
    - Severe cases may require joint aspiration.

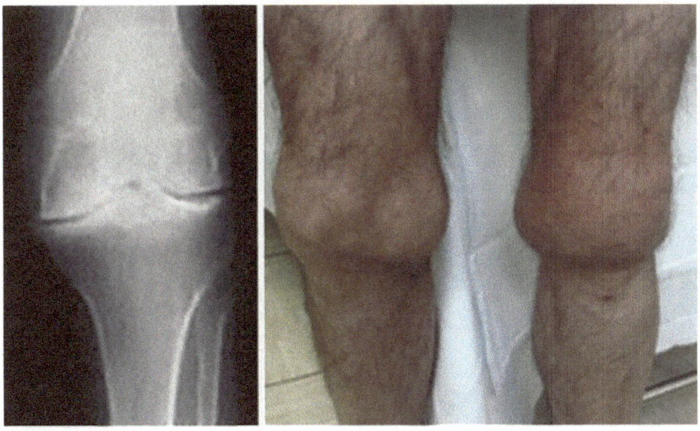

ALKAPTONURIA

Features

- Because of deficiency of homogentisate oxidase.
- *Characterized by:*
    - Ochronosis: Dark pigmentation of connective tissues (ear cartilage and sclera).
    - Calcification of cartilage.
    - Appearance of homogentisate in urine.
    - Urine turns dark on exposure to atmosphere.
- Vitamin C is given in treatment.

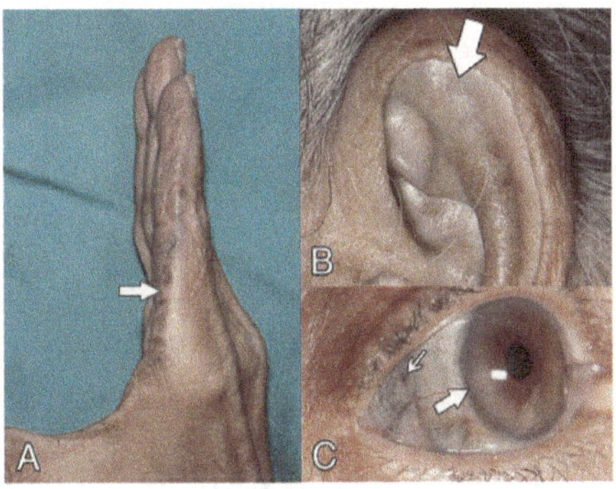

CHAPTER 8

PEDIATRIC ORTHOPEDICS

CONGENITAL TALIPES EQUINO VARUS/ CTEV

Features

- CTEV/clubfoot can be idiopathic or secondary.
- Idiopathic CTEV: Present since birth and there is no definitive cause.
- *Secondary CTEV:*
    - As the name suggest, it is due to:
        - Some paralytic disorder (polio, spina bifida).
        - Arthrogryposis multiplex congenita or.
        - Burns.
- *Clinical features:*
    - Size of foot and heel is small.
    - **Deformities** of foot are forefoot adduction, equinus, inversion (vowels: A, E, I), varus and tibial torsion.
    - Deep creases are noted on the medial side of sole and back of heel.
    - Lateral border of foot is gently convex.
- *Manipulation should begin:*
    - Immediately after birth by mother after every feed.
    - This should be carried out for a month till the skin is mature enough to tolerate the cast.
- *Corrective manipulation and casting:*
    - Done only after first month.
    - Ponseti method (serial casting) is **preferred**.
    - Correction is maintained in DB splint.

- *PMSTR (Postero-Medial Soft Tissue Release):*
  - Done at 2 years.
  - Child is grown up enough to tolerate anaesthesia and structures are well developed to be differentiated, otherwise one may cut a nerve mistaking it for a tendon.
- *Treatment of chronic neglected cases:*
  - **Triple** arthrodesis (Triple means three; arthrodesis means fusion of joint; it done after the age of 12 years after skeletal maturity, otherwise it is difficult to achieve fusion).
  - Joints fused are subtalar (talo-calcaneal), talo-navicular and calcaneo-cuboid (out of these three, talo-navicular joint is the difficult one to fuse).
- **Previously** Kite's method was used in which the deformities were corrected in the sequence of vowels **AIE** that is adduction, inversion and equinus, failing which rocker-bottom foot could have occurred.

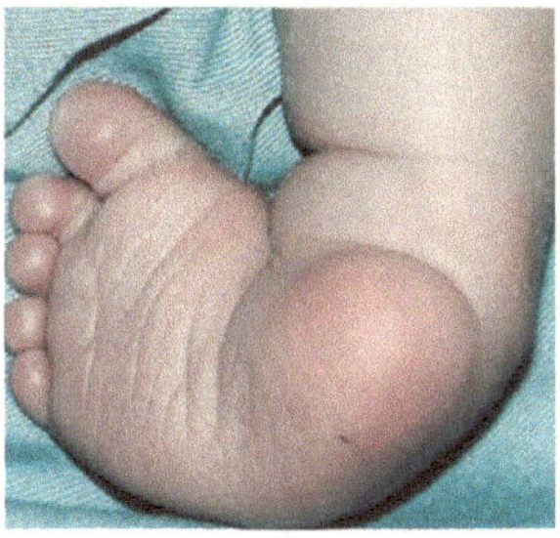

PERTHE'S DISEASE

Features

- Also known as coxa **plana**.
- Defined as: **Osteochondritis** of femoral head epiphysis.
- Here, the femoral head becomes partly or holly **avascular** and deformed.
- Due to recurrent episodes of **ischemia**.
- Affects boys in the age group of **5-10** years.
- Abduction is nearly always limited and internal rotation too.
- Investigation of **choice** for Perthes disease: MRI.
- Management aims at containment of femoral head within the acetabulum.

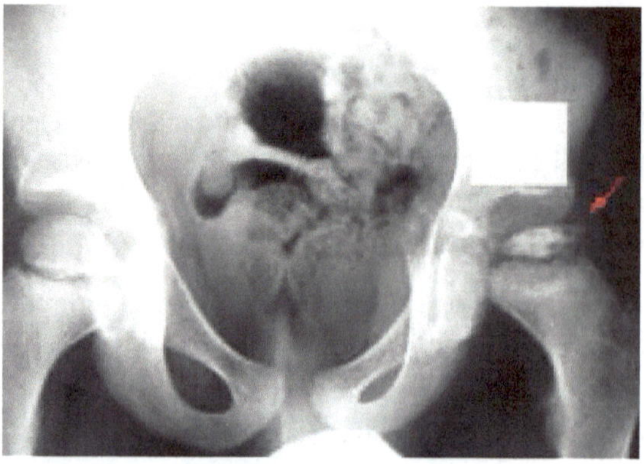

DEVELOPMENTAL DYSPLASIA OF HIP

Features

- Also known as congenital dislocation of the hip.
- *Screening tests:*
  - Ortolani's test.
  - Barlow's test.
- Limitation of abduction of hip.
- Abnormal waddling gait.
- Asymmetrical thigh folds.
- Galeazzi's sign.
- Telescopy test positive.

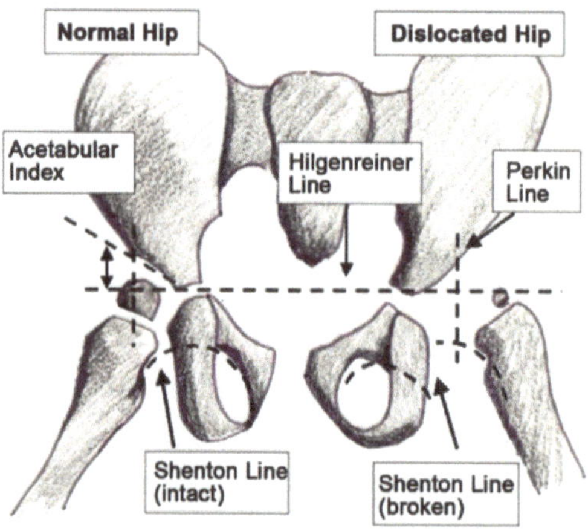

- *X-ray:*
    - Break in **Shenton's** line.
    - Upper femoral epiphysis lies on the outer aspect of the vertical line and above the horizontal line.
- *Treatment:*
    - Von-Rosen **splint** (1-6 months).
    - Acetabular reconstruction procedures (Pemberton's, Salter's, Chiari's etc.).

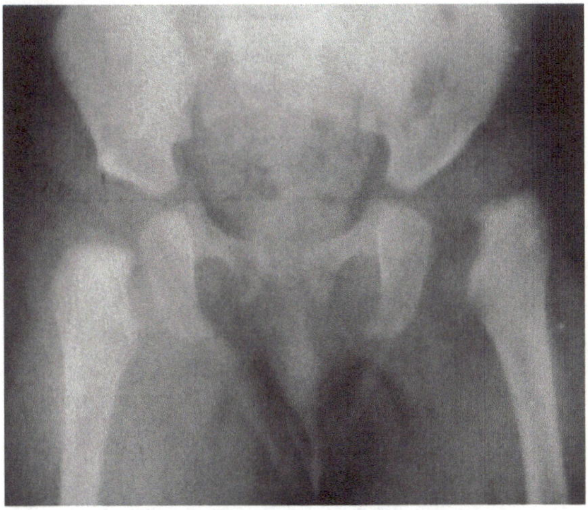

SLIPPED CAPITAL FEMORAL EPIPHYSIS

Features

- **Most commonly** affects male.
- Age: **10-16** years.
- Pain in the groin.
- *Limitation of:*
    - Internal rotation and
    - Abduction.
- Positive Trendelenburg's test.
- Positive **Trethowan's** sign on X-ray.
- Requires **prompt** surgical treatment.

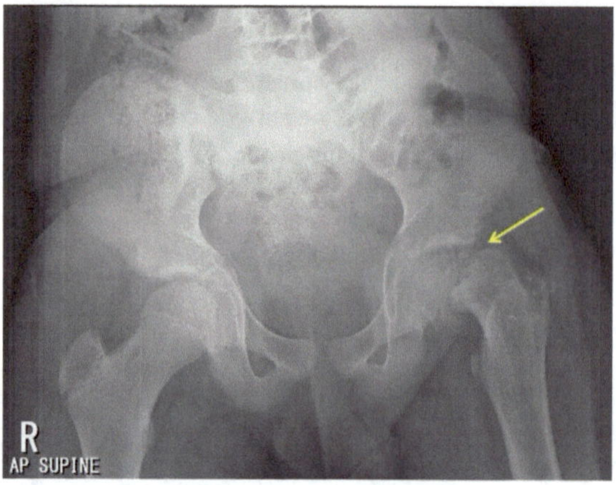

CONGENITAL/ INFANTILE TORTICOLLIS

Features

- Also known as wry neck.
- Due to fibrosis of sternocleidomastoid muscle and hence it fails to elongates as the child grows.

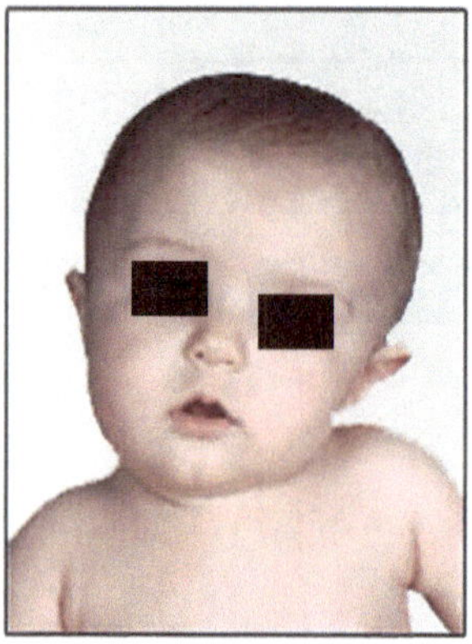

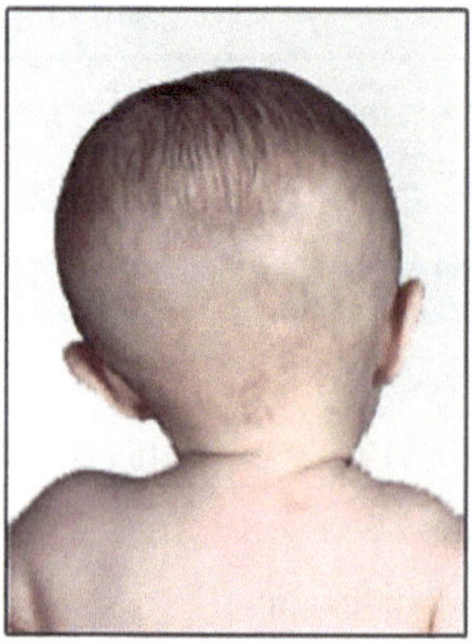

SPRENGEL'S SHOULDER

Features

- Also known as congenital high scapula.
- There is permanent elevation of the shoulder girdle and scapula lies high in position.

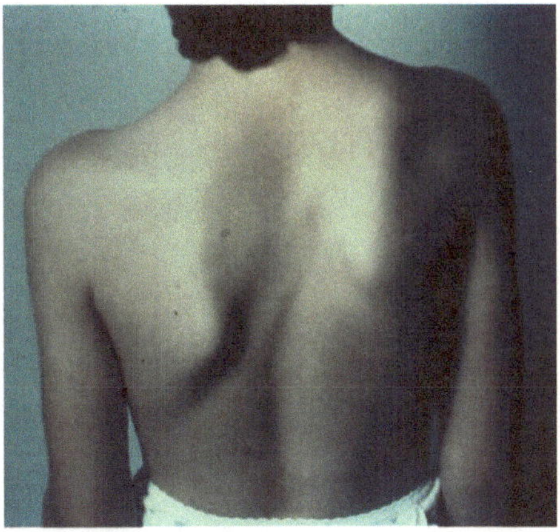

KLIPPEL-FEIL SYNDROME

Features

- There is congenital fusion of one or more of the cervical vertebrae
- Classical triad:
    - Short web neck.
    - Low hair line.
    - Restricted neck movements.

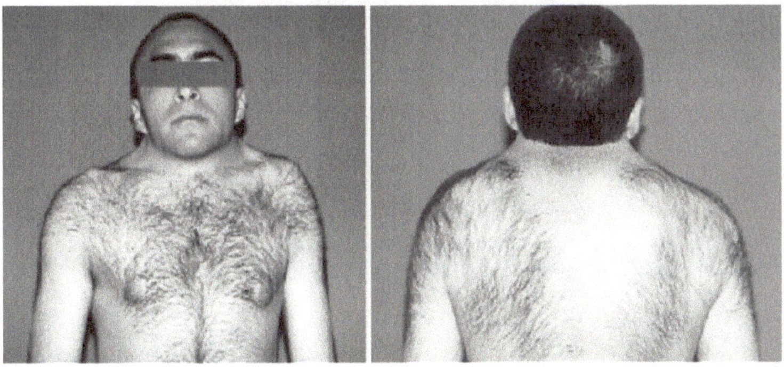

RADIAL CLUB HAND

Features

- Absent/deficiency of radius associated with inadequately developed thumb.

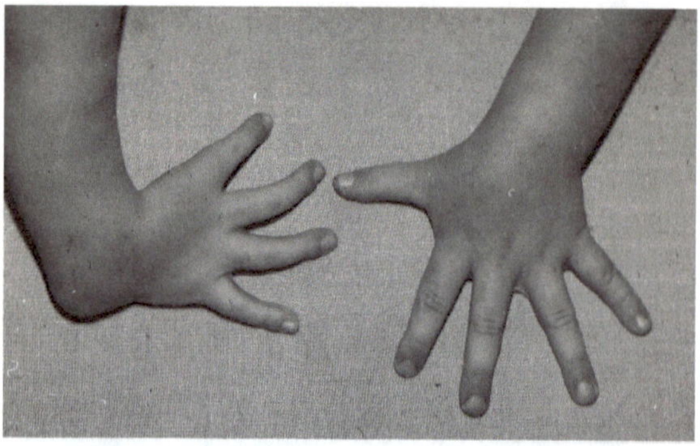

CONGENITAL PSEUDO-ARTHROSIS OF TIBIA

Features

- Seen mostly in the lower to middle third of the tibia with cupping of proximal bone end and pointing of distal bone end.
- Managed by Ilizarov fixator with bone grafting.

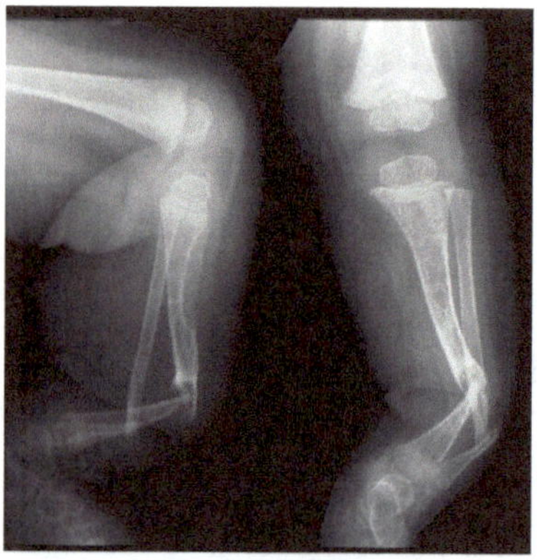

DUCHENNE MUSCULAR DYSTROPHY

Features

- X-linked recessive inheritance.
- Mutation in dystrophin gene.
- Weakness of proximal muscles.
- **Pseudohypertrophy** of calf muscles is seen.
- While getting up from the floor, patient climbs on himself (**Gower's** sign).

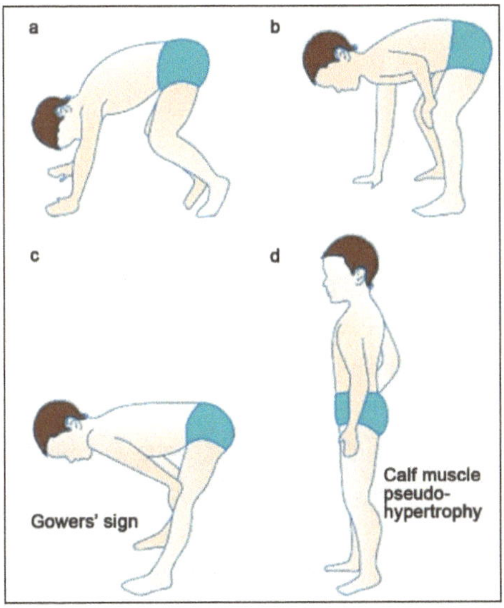

SCOLIOSIS

Scoliosis:

- *Braces used:*
  - Boston brace.
  - Milwaukee brace.
- *Radiological assessment:*
  - Cobb's angle (an angle drawn between the line passing through the margins of vertebrae at the ends of the primary and secondary curve).
- *Reisser's sign:*
  - Iliac apophysis fuses with the iliac bone at skeletal maturity and marks the completion of growth.
  - This indicates that there is **no** possibility of curve worsening further.

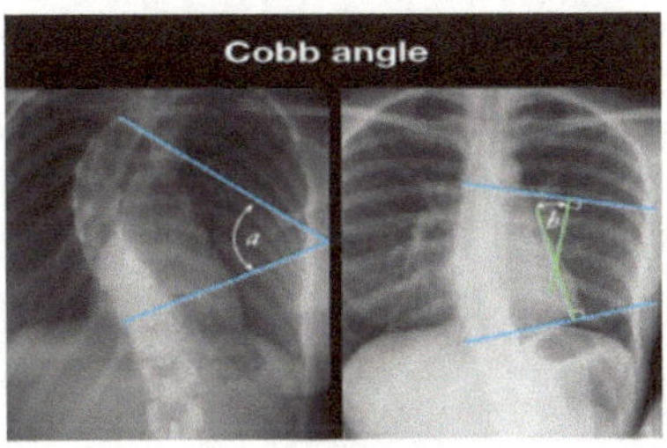

GREEN-STICK FRACTURE

Features

- Incomplete fracture, seen only in children.
- Cortex in tension fracture completely.
- Fracture in compression remains intact.
- Fracture-line looks like a broken green stick, which does not break completely in two separate pieces.
- While managing such fractures, the fracture has to be completed first on the intact side.

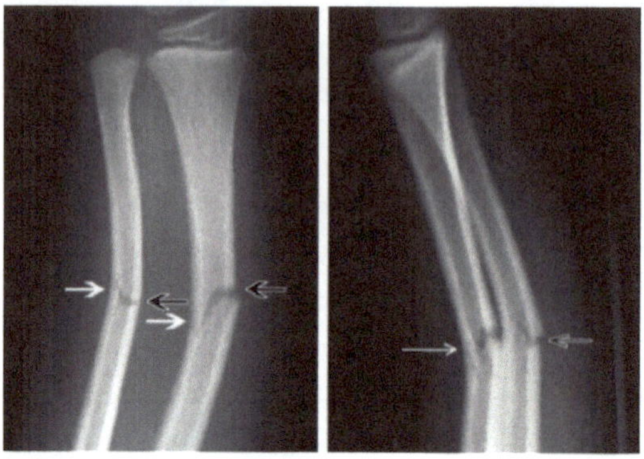

TORUS/ BUCKLE FRACTURE

Features

- Resembles the base of an architectural column.
- Usually occurs at the site of transition from diaphysis to metaphysis.

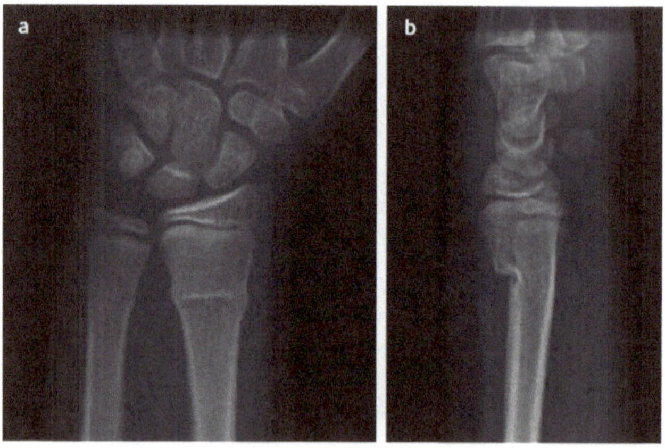

EPIPHYSEAL INJURIES

Features

- Classified as per Salter & Harris classification.
- Thurston Holland fragment/sign is seen in type II.

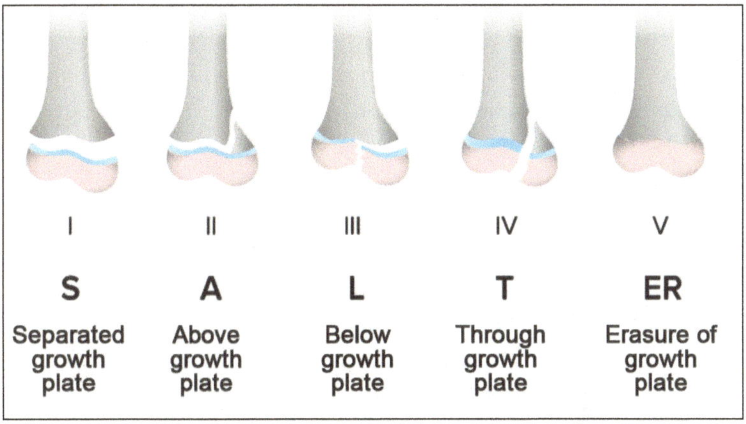

CHAPTER 9

BASICS OF TRAUMATOLOGY

FRACTURE AND EPONYMS

Fractures & eponyms:

- *Greenstick fracture:*
  - Childrens.
  - Bending force.
  - Distraction of cortex on convex side & compression on the concave side (cortex intact).
- Bennet's fracture: Intra-articular base of 1st metacarpal.
- Rolando's fracture: Intra-articular fracture base of first metacarpal with comminution.
- Jefferson's fracture: Burst fracture of C1 (atlas).
- Hangman's fracture: Traumatic spondylolisthesis of cervical vertebrae 2.
- Monteggia fracture: Proximal ulna fracture with dislocation of proximal superior radio-ulnar joint.
- Galeazzi fracture: Galeazzi is fracture distal radius with dislocation of distal radio-ulnar joint.
- March fracture: Stress fracture of shaft of 2nd or 3rd metatarsal (commonly).
- Pott's fracture: Bimalleolar fracture.

MOST COMMON IN FRACTURES

Most common:

- Bone fractured in body: Clavicle.
- Bone fractured during birth: Clavicle.

FRACTURE CLASSIFICATION

Features

- Open fracture: There is a wound and the fracture hematoma is communicating with external environment.
- Closed fracture: Overlying skin and tissues are intact (over a fracture).
- Pathological fracture: Bone has been weakened by some local or systemic condition and it then fractures with minimal trauma.

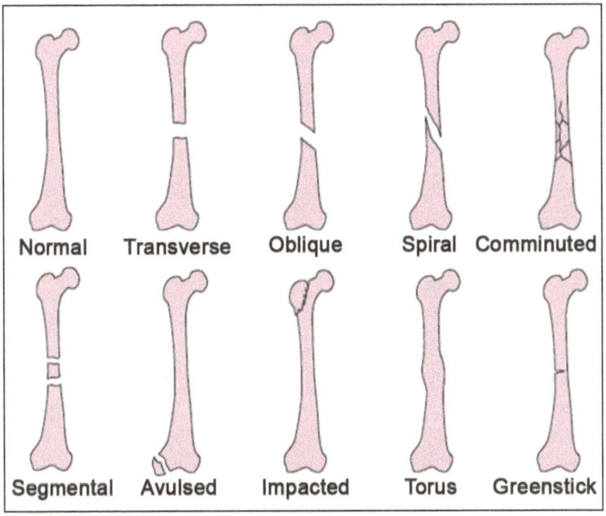

FRACTURE HEALING

Features

- Most important factor for fracture healing: Degree of immobilization
- *Stages in fracture healing:*
    - Hematoma (<1 week)
    - Granulation tissue (2-3 weeks)
    - Callus formation (4-12 weeks)
    - Remodelling (1-2 years)
    - Modelling (>2 years)

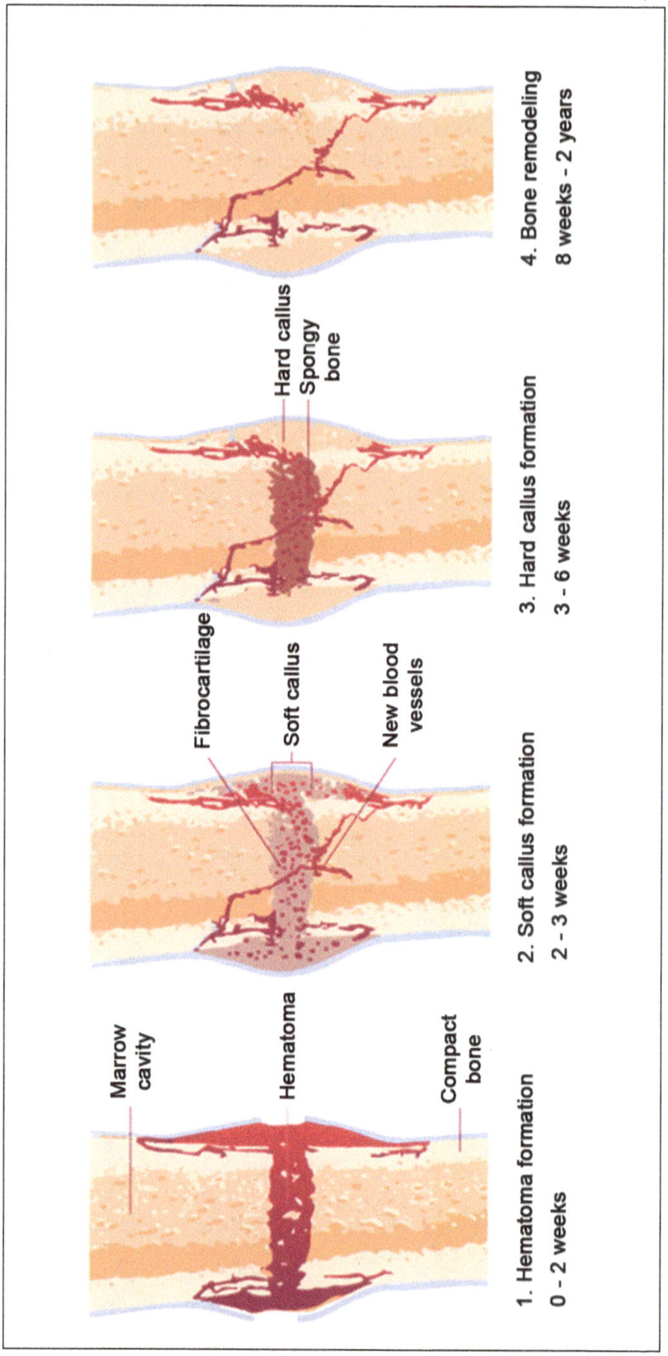
Marrow cavity
Hematoma
Compact bone
1. Hematoma formation
0 - 2 weeks
Fibrocartilage
Soft callus
New blood vessels
2. Soft callus formation
2 - 3 weeks
Hard callus
Spongy bone
3. Hard callus formation
3 - 6 weeks
4. Bone remodeling
8 weeks - 2 years

DELAYED UNION

Features

- Fracture is in process of union but is taking more time than the usual

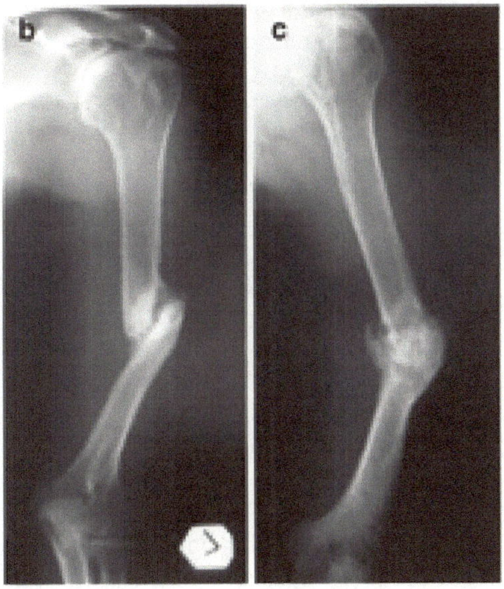

MALUNION

Features

- Fracture has united but in a wrong position
- Usually seen with intertrochanteric fracture femur, fracture Colle's etc.

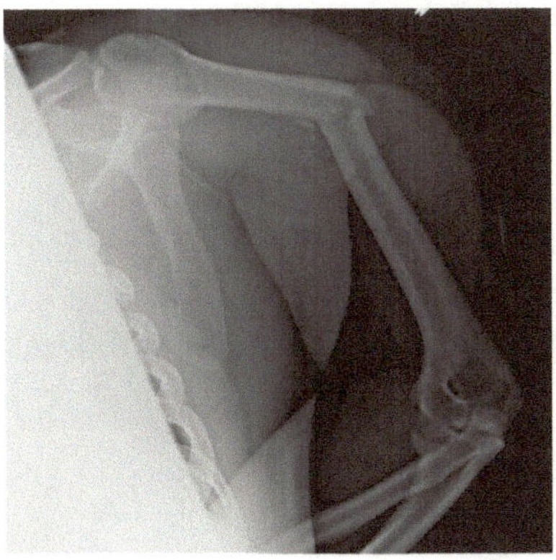

NON-UNION

Features

- Fracture has not united at the end of 9 months (This time limit rule is not applicable for fracture neck of femur)

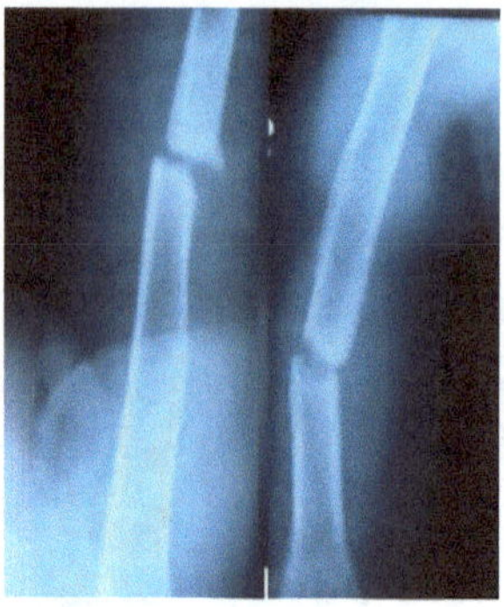

COMPARTMENT SYNDROME

Features

- Muscles are enclosed in an inelastic fascial compartment. If there is edema, it will compress muscles, which will lead to further edema and a vicious cycle continues.
- This can be encountered in **forearm and leg region** particularly after injury and a tight cast application.
- *Compartment syndrome is commonly seen in:*
    - Fracture supracondylar humerus (artery involved is brachial artery)
    - Fracture of proximal tibia
- **Most important sign** of Volkmann ischemia/ compartment syndrome: Passive stretch pain (when the fingers/ toes are stretched dorsally).
- In posterior compartment syndrome in leg region, toe dorsiflexion will cause pain
- Pulse is NOT a reliable indicator of compartment syndrome
- *Muscles commonly affected in forearm:*
    - Flexor digitorum profundus,
    - Flexor pollicis longus

- *Management:*
  - If this is because of a tight cast, bivalve it or remove it
  - In cases of impending compartment syndrome, one has to release the pressure on muscles by doing **fasciotomy**.
  - Structures cut during fasciotomy:
    - Skin
    - Superficial fascia
    - Subcutaneous fat
    - Deep fascia
    - Muscles are **NOT** cut

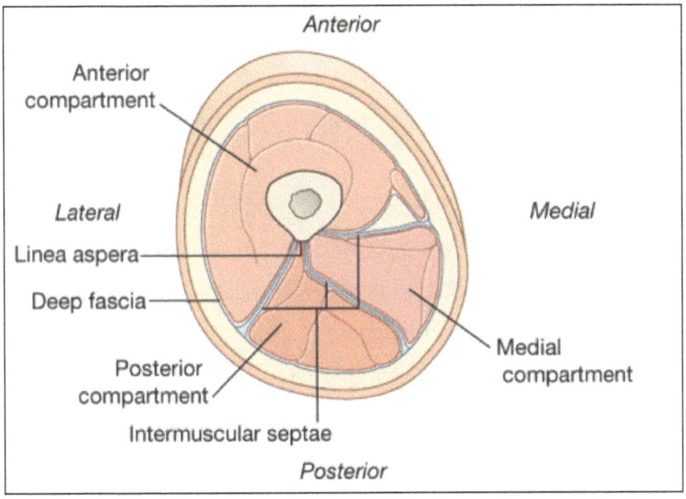

MYOSITIS OSSIFICANS

Features

- Heterotopic calcification and ossification in muscle tissue
- Mature bone is seen at periphery
- Commonly follows injury and massage
- **Most commonly** seen around elbow joint > hip joint
- **Most commonly** seen in brachialis muscle
- *Treatment:*
  - Acute cases: Immobilization

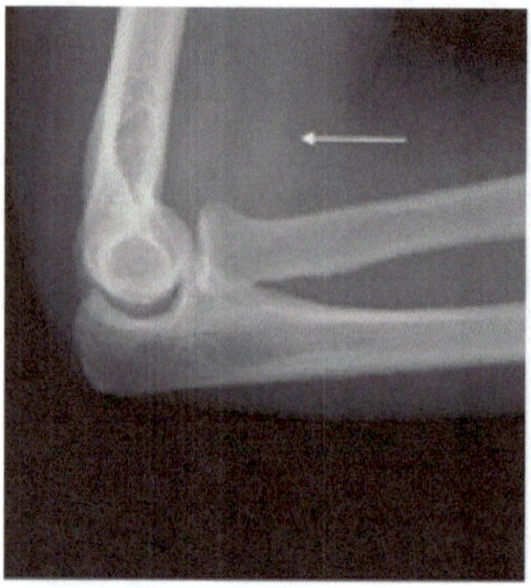

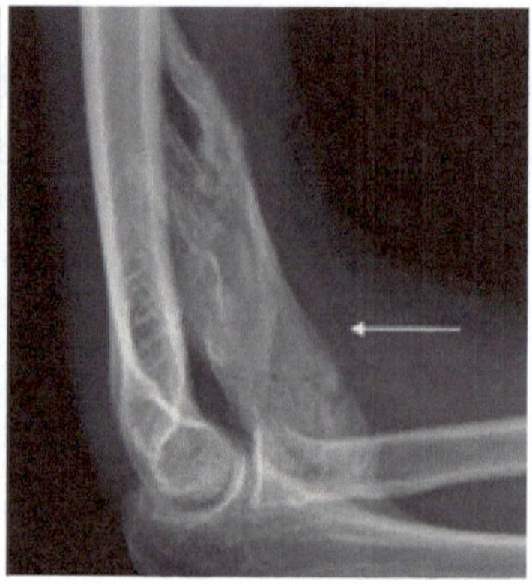

FAT EMBOLISM

Features

- *Early warning signs:*
    - Tachycardia
    - Slight hyperthermia
- *Classic triad* ***(Mnemonic: PNR)***:
    - **P**etechial rash in conjunctiva of lower eyelid, axilla, neck etc.
    - **N**eurological: Disorientation
    - **R**espiratory: Tachypnea/ dyspnea
- Aim of management is to maintain adequate oxygen level

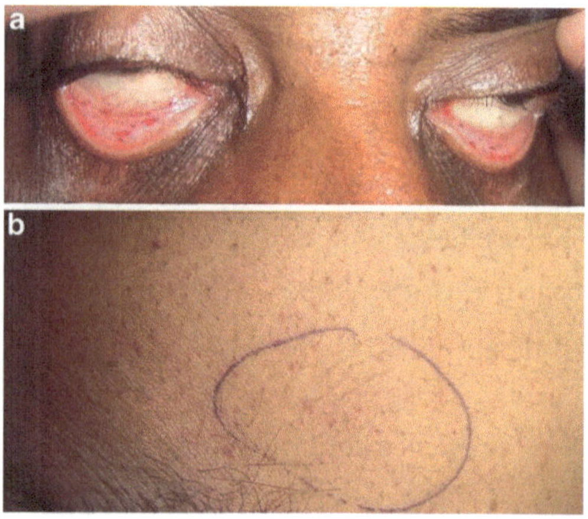

CHAPTER 10

MISCELLANEOUS TOPICS

OSTEOCHONDRITIS

Osteochondritis of bones & clinical conditions:

- Lunate: Kienbock's disease.
- Navicular: Kohler's disease.
- Tibial tuberosity: Osgood-Schlatter disease.
- Calcaneum: Sever's disease.
- Capitellum: Panner's disease.
- Thoracic spine: Scheuermann's disease.
- Metatarsal: Frieberg disease.

PAINFUL ARC SYNDROME

Features

- Painful arc syndrome is a clinical syndrome in which there is pain in the shoulder and upper arm during the mid-range of glenohumeral abduction.
- *Causes:*
    - Minor tears of the supraspinatus tendon.
    - Supraspinatus tendinitis.
    - Calcification of supraspinatus tendon.
    - Subacromial bursitis.
    - Fracture of the greater tuberosity.
- In all these conditions, the space between the upper end of the humerus and the acromion gets compromised, so that during mid-abduction the tendon of the rotator cuff gets nipped between the greater tuberosity and acromion.
- Affects middle aged and old people.
- Predominantly males.
- Localized tenderness at insertion of supraspinatus tendon.

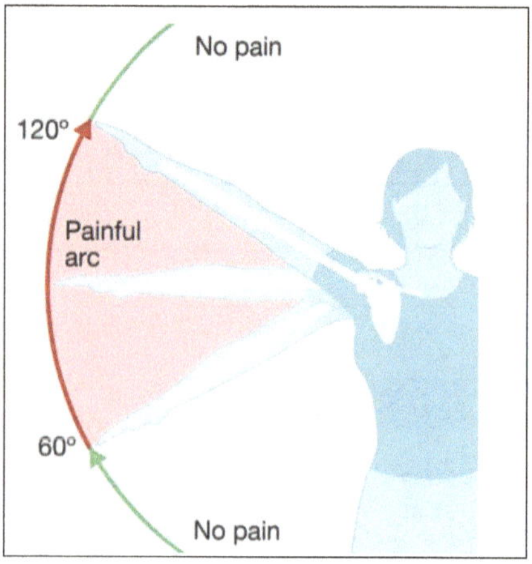

BURSITIS

Bursa inflamed and clinical conditions:

- Infrapatellar bursitis: Clergyman's knee.
- Prepatellar bursitis: Housemaid's knee.
- Olecranon bursitis: Student's elbow.

CASTS & USES

Casts and fractures in which they are used:

- Tube/Cylindrical cast: Knee fracture.
- Cast in glass holding position: Scaphoid fracture.
- PTB (Patellar tendon bearing) cast: Tibial fracture.

SPLINTS & USES

Splints and the conditions in which they are used:

- Von Rosen splint: CDH/ DDH (Developmental dysplasia of hip).
- Knuckle bender splint: Ulnar nerve palsy.
- Cock-up splint: Radial nerve palsy.
- Thomas splint: Fracture femur – anywhere.
- Bohler Braun splint: Fracture femur – anywhere.
- Dennis Brown splint: CTEV.
- Aeroplane splint: Brachial plexus injury.

SECTION 2

SELF-ASSESSMENT

{IMAGE BASED MCQs, CLINICAL MCQs and MCQs POINTS (One-liners)}

IMAGE BASED MCQs

1. A young patient presented with multiple swellings in the hand. X-ray is shown below. Most likely diagnosis:

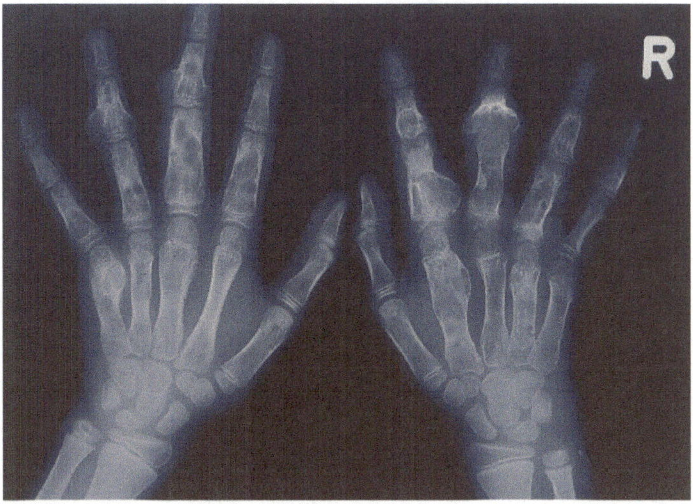

(a) Polyostotic fibrous dysplasia

(b) Multiple Enchondromatosis

(c) Multiple brown tumours

(d) Multiple exostosis

X-ray shows enchondroma.

Enchondromas comprise lobules of mature hyaline cartilage which are partially or completely encased by surrounding normal bone.

Small bones of the hands and feet are the commonest site of enchondroma, which is a benign tumour consisting of lobulated mass of cartilage encapsulated by fibrous tissue.

Answer: B i.e., Multiple enchondromatosis

2. **Identify the injury and the procedure done:**

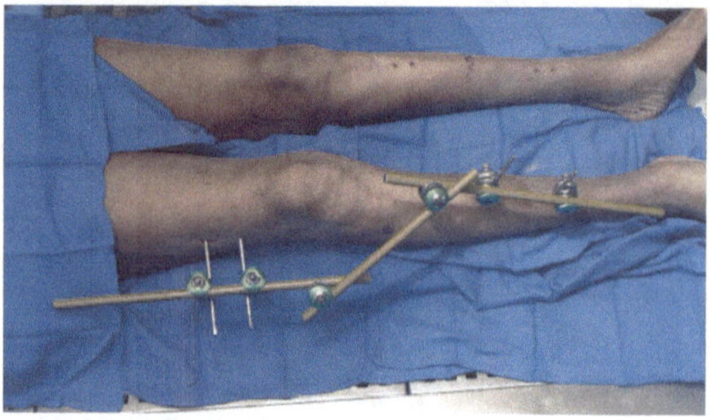

(a) Open fracture patella, Ilizarov fixator

(b) Fracture shaft of tibia; Spanning fixator

(c) Periarticular fracture of the knee; Spanning fixator

(d) Fracture shaft of femur; Spanning fixator

Image shows a knee-spanning external fixator.

A joint-spanning/spanning external fixator is fixed to femur and the tibia while the fracture zone (around knee joint) is left untouched.

Periarticular fracture of the knee is defined as a fracture occurring anywhere between the distal femur and the proximal tibia.

Answer: C i.e., Periarticular fracture zof the knee; Spanning fixator

3. **What would be the best management plan for the injury shown below in the X-ray?**

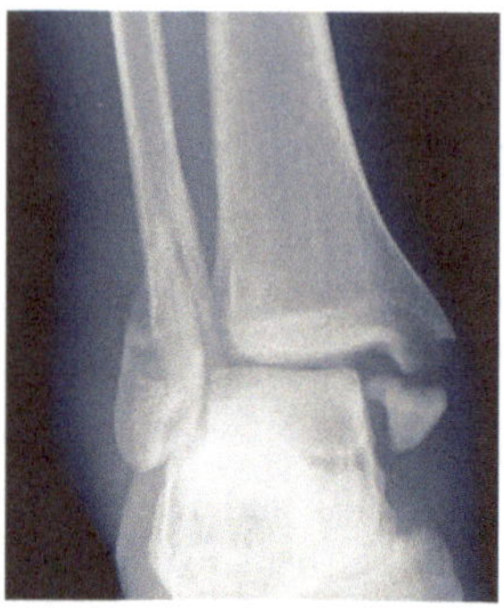

(a) Analgesic, Operative fixation

(b) Analgesic, Closed reduction, Cast

(c) Analgesic, Bed rest

(d) Analgesic, Neurological assessment

X-ray shows displaced bimalleolar fracture and is best managed operatively in an adult.

A bimalleolar fracture is a fracture of the lateral malleolus and the medial malleolus.

Answer: A i.e., Analgesic, Operative fixation

4. **A young adult presented to Orthopedic clinic with the complaints of pain and swelling over the radial aspect of the wrist following a fall on out-stretched hand. Treating doctor noticed tenderness in anatomical snuffbox and applied a cast as shown in the figure. Which bone is fractured in the given patient?**

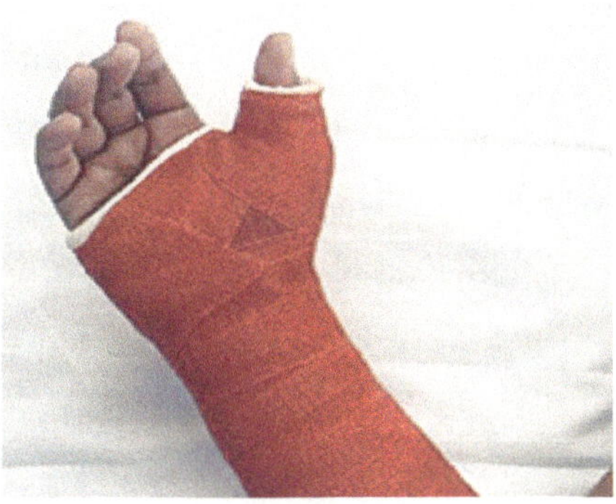

(a) Lower end of radius

(b) Scaphoid

(c) Base of first metacarpal

(d) Ulnar styloid process

Clinical presentation and image are indicative of fracture scaphoid.

Scaphoid Fractures are the most common carpal bone *fracture*, often occurring after a fall onto an outstretched hand.

Image shows a cast applied in glass holding position, in which the wrist is maintained in a little dorsiflexion and radial deviation. Such a cast is applied for fractures of scaphoid.

Answer: B i.e., Scaphoid

5. **Study the X-ray of the ankle joint of a diabetic patient. Most likely diagnosis:**

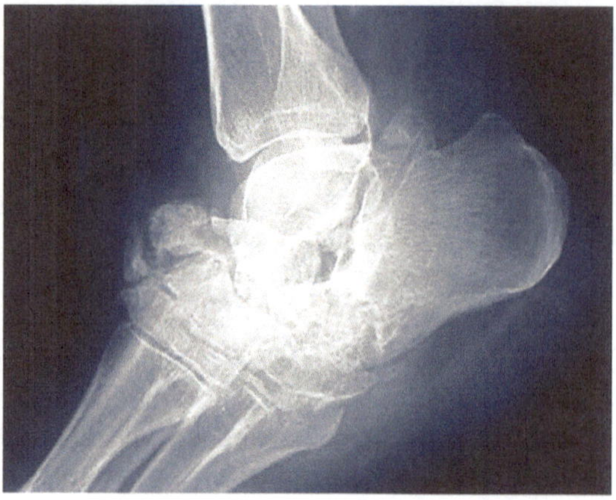

(a) Osteomyelitis of calcaneum (b) Calcaneal spur

(c) Charcot joint (d) Gouty arthritis

Answer: C. Charcot joint

6. **Which nerve palsy can result in this kind of appearance?**

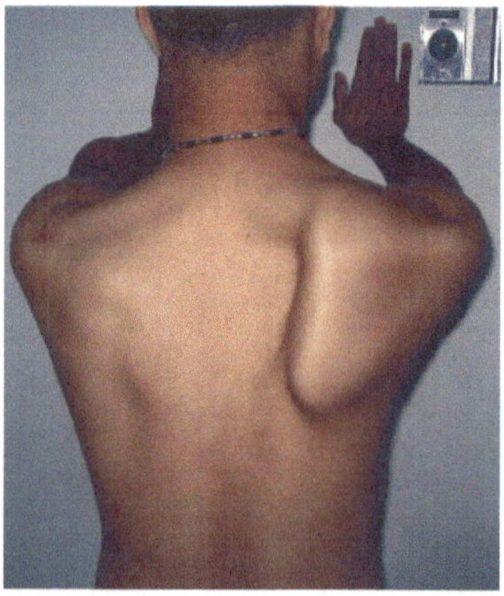

(a) Long thoracic nerve (b) Thoracodorsal nerve

(c) Suprascapular nerve (d) Subscapular nerve

The serratus anterior muscle can be examined by asking the patient to push against a wall with both hands. The medial border of the scapula on the affected side will become prominent (winging of scapula). Serratus anterior muscle is supplied by long thoracic nerve.

Answer: A i.e., Long thoracic nerve

7. **Which nerve is injured?**

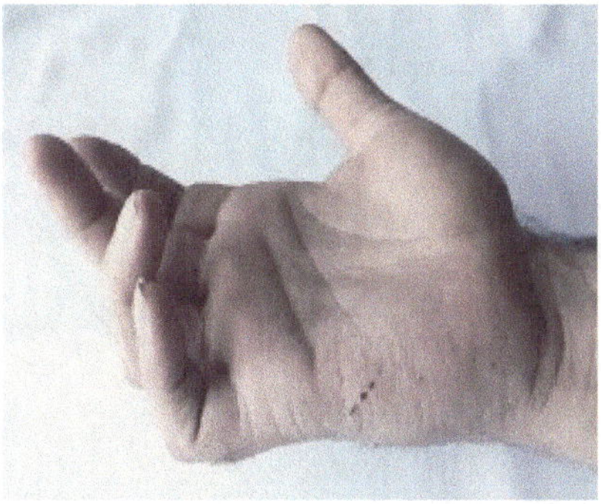

(a) Radial nerve (b) Median nerve

(c) Ulnar nerve (d) Ulnar + median nerve

In ulnar nerve palsy, only the medial two fingers develop clawing while all the four fingers develop clawing in combined median and ulnar nerve palsies. Clawing may not become apparent in the early post-injury period.

Answer: C i.e., Ulnar nerve

8. **Identify the condition shown below in a known case of rheumatoid arthritis:**

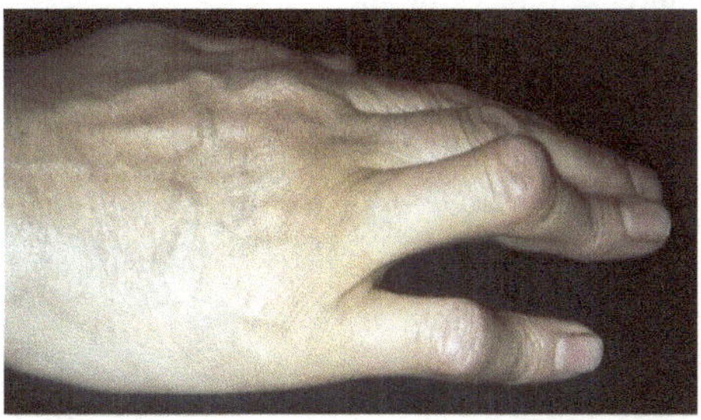

(a) Mallet finger (b) Swan neck deformity

(c) Boutonniere deformity (d) Dupuytren's contracture

Answer: C. Boutonniere deformity

9. **A 25 years old male presented to the Orthopedic OPD with the complaints of swelling and vague pain around the wrist area. On examination, an eccentric, bony swelling was found. Surface of the swelling was smooth. X-ray of the patient is shown below. Most likely diagnosis:**

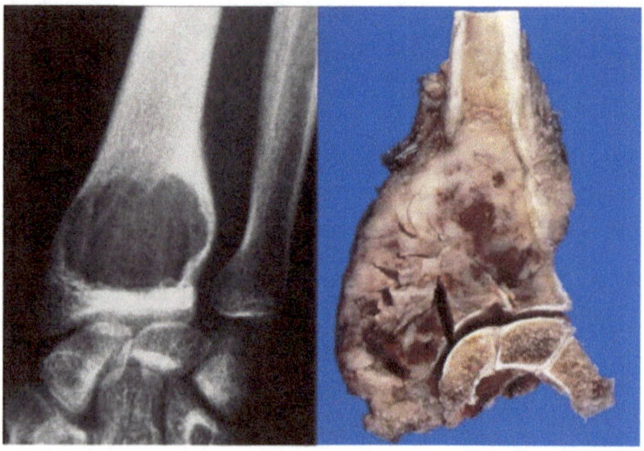

(a) Ewing sarcoma (b) Giant cell tumour
(c) Osteosarcoma (d) Metastasis

Clinical presentation and image are indicative of giant cell tumour.

A giant cell tumor is a rare, aggressive non-cancerous tumor. It usually develops near a joint at the end of the bone.

On X-ray, there is a solitary, lytic lesion, eccentric in location, with expansion of the overlying cortex, and soap-bubble appearance (tumour is homogenously lytic with trabecula of the remnants of bone traversing it, giving rise to a loculated appearance). There is no calcification within the tumour.

Answer: B i.e., Giant cell tumour

10. **A 1 month old baby was brought to the Orthopedic OPD with the foot deformity as shown in the image. What is the best management of such a case:**

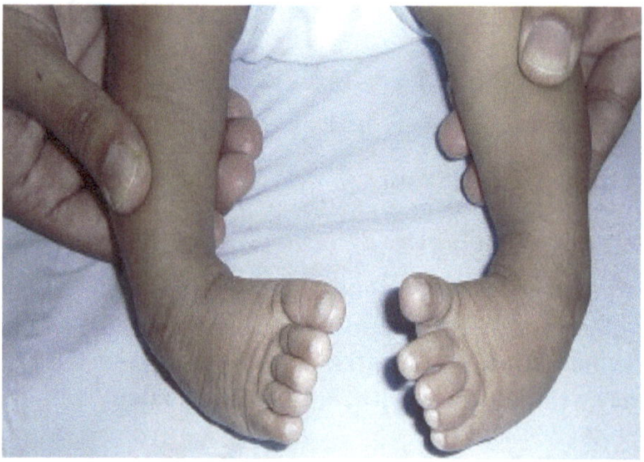

(a) Manipulation and serial casting

(b) Postero-Medial SOft Tissue Release/ PMSTR

(c) Dilwyn-Evan's procedure

(d) Triple arthrodesis

Image shows CTEV.

Congenital talipes equinovarus (CTEV), is often known as 'club-foot'. It is defined as fixation of the foot in adduction, in supination and in varus, i.e., inclined inwards, axially rotated outwards and pointing downwards.

Manipulation and serial corrective casting by Ponseti's technique is the preferred method for CTEV in a newborn. Treatment is started within 1st week of life.

Answer: A i.e., Manipulation and serial casting

11. Make a clinical diagnosis:

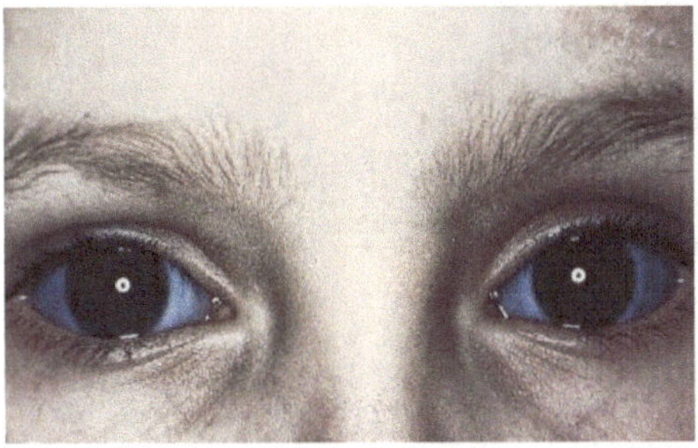

(a) Paget's disease

(b) Rickets

(c) Scurvy

(d) Osteogenesis imperfecta

Answer: D. Osteogenesis imperfecta

12. Identify the bone fractured in the given image:

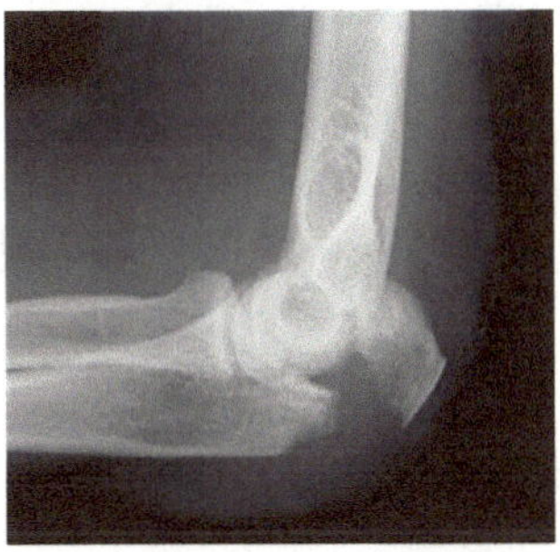

(a) Head of radius (b) Capitellum

(c) Olecranon process (d) Trochlea

X-ray shows fracture olecranon process (of ulna).

Olecranon Fractures are common *fractures* of the elbow that lead to loss of extensor mechanism.

Fracture olecranon is managed by TBW (tension band wiring)

Answer: C i.e., Olecranon process

13. Identify the fracture:

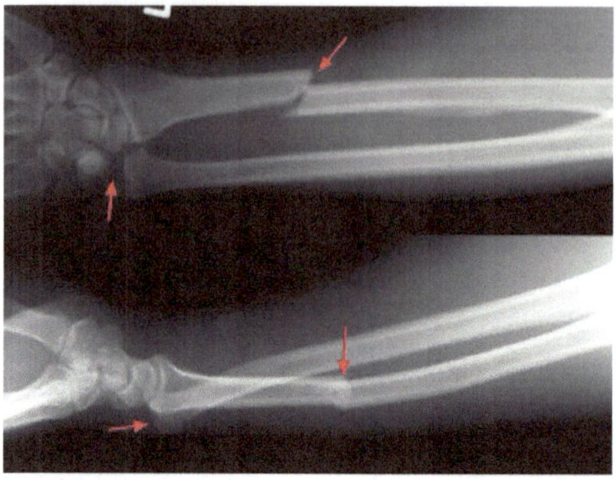

(a) Colle's fracture (b) Monteggia fracture

(c) Galeazzi fracture (d) Smith's fracture

X-ray shows Galeazzi fracture dislocation.

Galeazzi fracture dislocation involves fracture of lower third of radius and dislocation/ subluxation of the inferior radio-ulnar joint.

Answer: C i.e., Galeazzi fracture

14. A male child developed right sided limp few days after his third birthday. There was no history of injury. He was reviewed by a pediatric orthopedician within 48 hours of onset of the limp. On examination, there was fever and vitals were stable. Child was having an antalgic gait with a lurch towards right side but there was full range of movements at both hip and knee. There was no pain during movement. ESR was raised but all other blood tests (total leucocyte count, C-reactive protein and calcium profile) were normal. X-ray pelvis with hip joints is shown below. Most likely diagnosis:

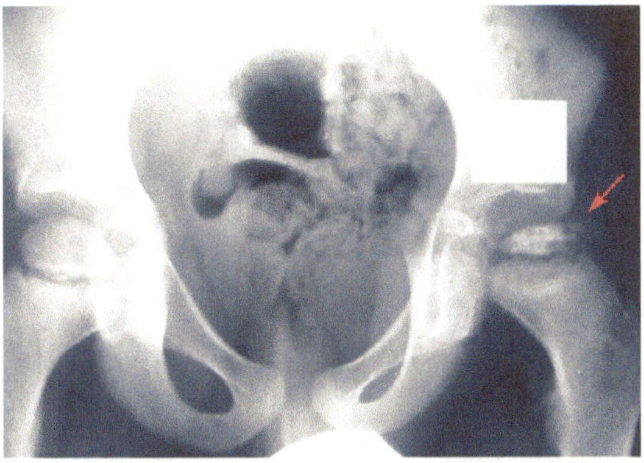

(a) Gaucher's disease (b) Rickets

(c) Scurvy (d) Perthe's disease

Answer: D. Perthe's disease

15. **Study the X-ray and make a clinical diagnosis:**

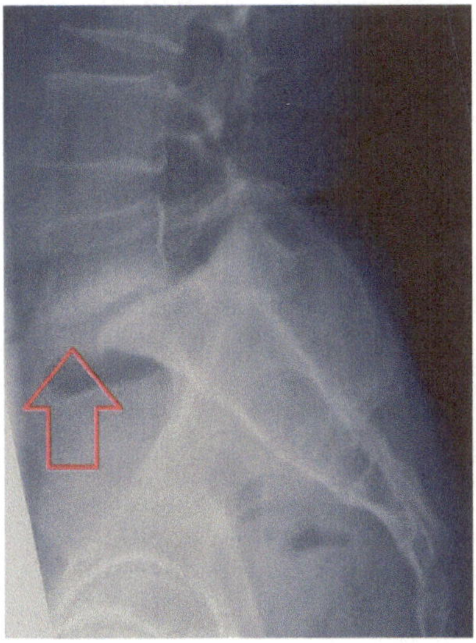

(a) Ankylosing spondylitis

(b) Retrolisthesis

(c) Spondylolisthesis

(d) Wedge fracture lumbar vertebrae

Answer: C. Spondylolisthesis

16. **A patient sustained injury over the hip in a RTA. Mechanism of injury impacts on the knee when the knee and hip were flexed and the hip was adducted. X-ray pelvis with both the hips was done as shown below. Which nerve is likely to get injured 2:**

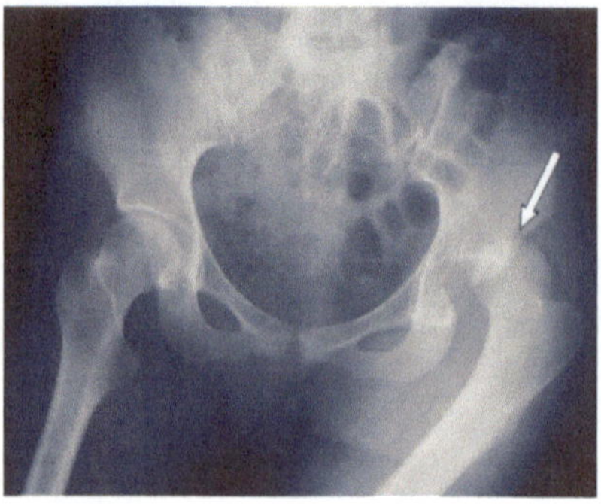

(a) Femoral nerve

(b) Sciatic nerve

(c) Lateral cutaneous nerve of thigh

(d) Obturator nerve

Clinical presentation and X-ray are indicative of posterior dislocation of the hip joint.

Answer: B. Sciatic nerve

17. **Splint shown in the figure is used for:**

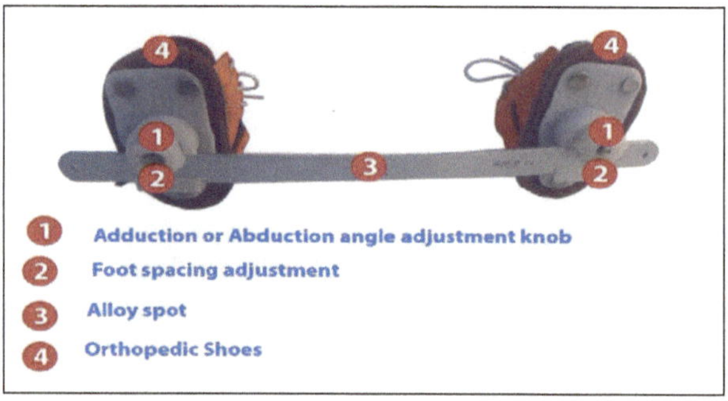

(a) Slipped capital femoral epiphyses

(b) Perthe's disease

(c) CTEV

(d) Congenital hip dislocation

Image shows DB splint.

Dennis Brown splint is used for maintenance of correction achieved by serial casting in CTEV.

Answer: C i.e., CTEV

18. **A young male had a road traffic accident. His lower limb was in an attitude of flexion, adduction & internal rotation. X-ray was done, which is shown below. Which nerve injury is most likely to occur in such a case?**

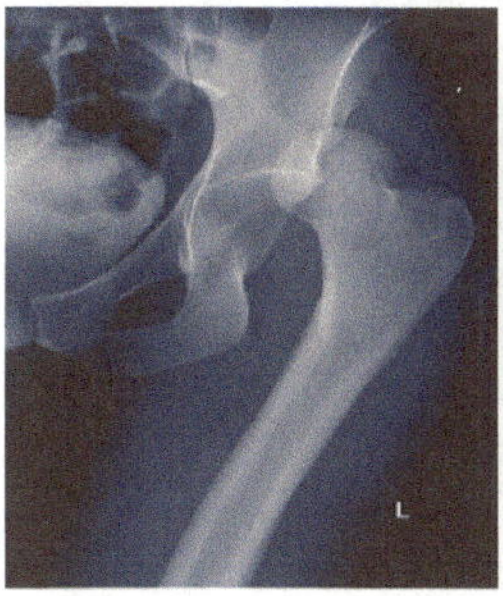

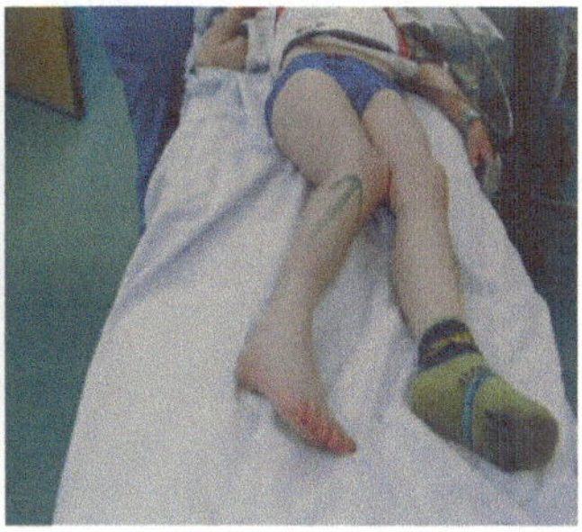

(a) Common peroneal nerve (b) Obturator nerve

(c) Sciatic nerve (d) Femoral nerve

Clinical presentation and image are indicative of posterior dislocation of the hip joint.

Posterior hip dislocations are the most common type and are reduced by placing longitudinal traction with internal rotation on the *hip*.

Sciatic nerve may be injured.

Answer: C i.e., Sciatic nerve

19. **Identify the brace shown:**

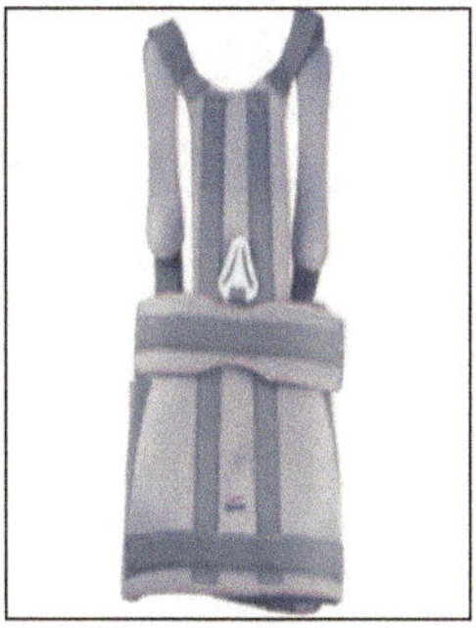

(a) Milwaukee brace
(b) Taylor's brace
(c) ASH brace
(d) Lumbar corset

Answer: B. Taylor's brace

20. Which bone is fractured in the given X-ray?

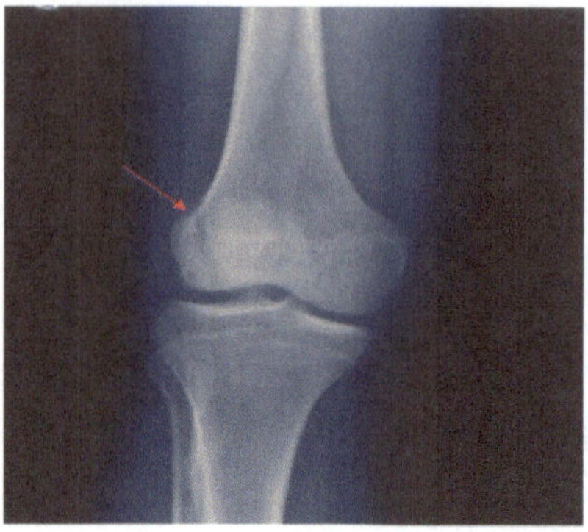

(a) Femoral shaft
(b) Femoral condyles
(c) Patella
(d) Tibial condyles

Answer: C. Patella

21. Which nerve can be injured in the type of humerus fracture shown below?

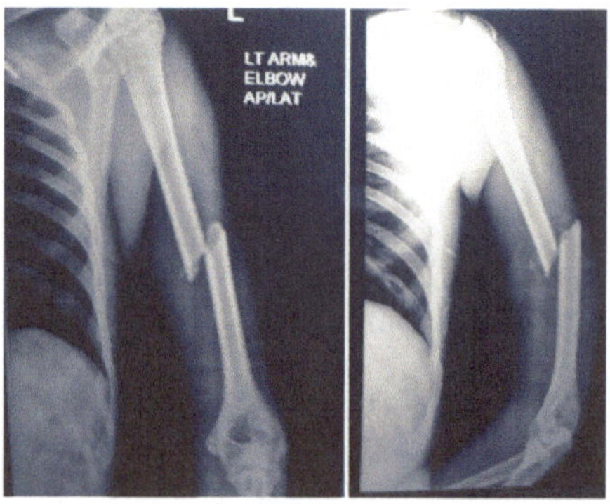

(a) Radial nerve
(b) Median nerve
(c) Ulnar nerve
(d) Musculocutaneous nerve

X-ray shows fracture shaft of the humerus.

Answer: A i.e., Radial nerve

22. Identify the given prosthesis:

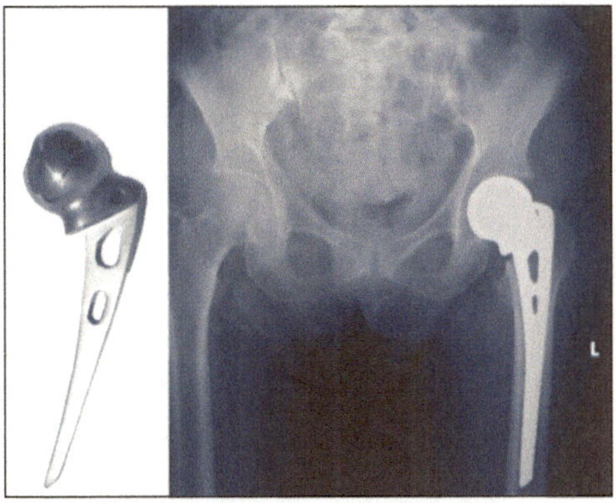

(a) Austin Moore prosthesis

(b) Thompson prosthesis

(c) Bipolar prosthesis

(d) Total hip replacement prosthesis

Austin-Moore prosthesis is used in hemi-replacement arthroplasty of hip (replacement of femoral head), following fracture neck of femur in elderly.

Answer: A i.e., Austin Moore prosthesis

23. Identify the condition shown in the X-ray below:

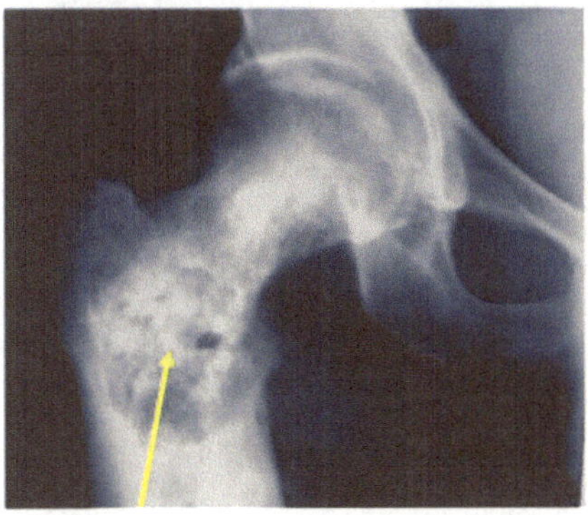

(a) Ewing sarcoma

(b) Chondrosarcoma

(c) Osteosarcoma

(d) Osteochondroma

Answer: B. Chondrosarcoma

24. A male had a short neck, low posterior hairline and reduced neck movements. X-ray showed apparent fusion of the cervical vertebrae. Clinical picture is shown below. Most likely diagnosis:

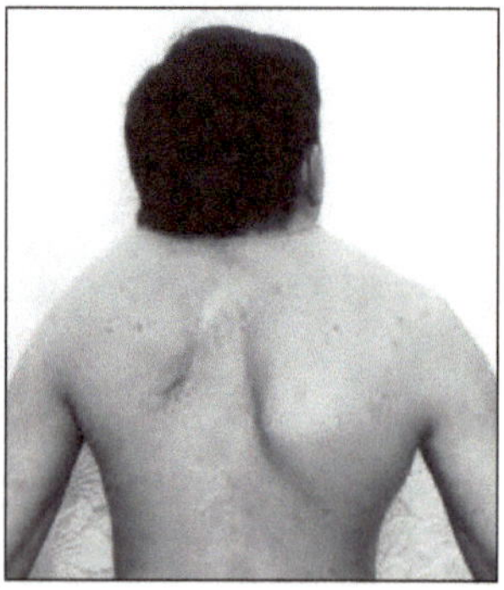

(a) Sprengel shoulder
(b) Torticollis
(c) Klippel Feil syndrome
(d) Scoliosis

Answer: C. Klippel Feil syndrome

25. A 20 years male presented with gradual onset of backache and morning stiffness since last 6 months. He also noticed redness in the eyes. X-ray was done as shown below. Most likely diagnosis:

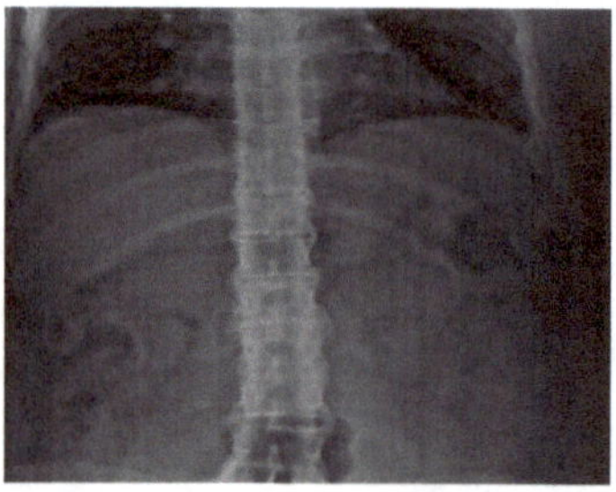

(a) Spondylitis
(b) Tuberculosis of spine
(c) Ankylosing spondylitis
(d) Alkaptonuria

Clinical presentation and image are indicative of ankylosing spondylitis.

Ankylosing spondylitis (AS) is a chronic, inflammatory disease of the axial spine. Chronic back pain and progressive spinal stiffness are the common symptoms.

X-ray shows bamboo spine.

Redness in eyes suggest acute anterior uveitis.

Answer: C i.e., Ankylosing spondylitis

26. A 4 years old child presented with lassitude, anemia and painful limbs. X-ray showed the presence of dense white lines as shown below. Most likely diagnosis:

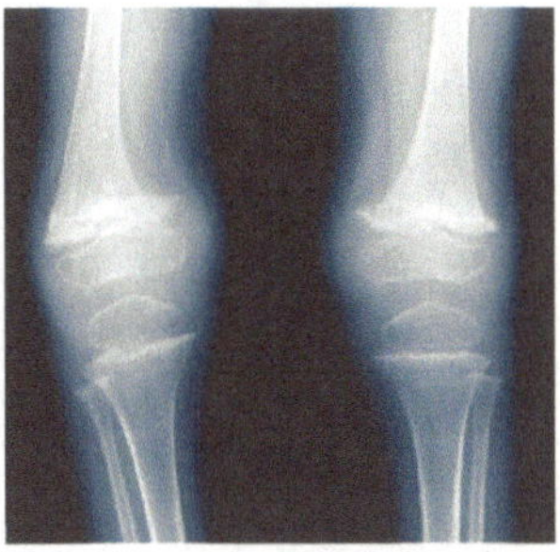

(a) Rickets (b) Scurvy

(c) Osteomalacia (d) Osteoporosis

Clinical presentation and images are indicative of scurvy.

Scurvy is a disease that occurs when there is severe lack of vitamin C (ascorbic acid) in diet. Scurvy causes general weakness, anemia, gum disease, and skin hemorrhages.

Dense white lines in the X-ray are white line of Frenkel.

Answer: B i.e., Scurvy

27. Which of the following condition is managed in the way as shown in the image:

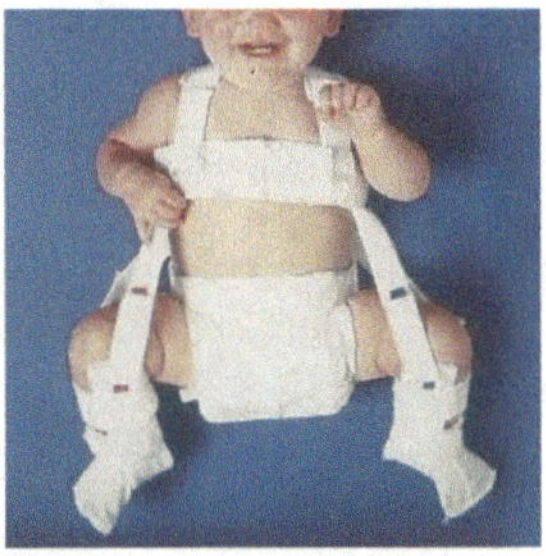

(a) Developmental dysplasia of the hip

(b) Slipped capital femoral epiphyses

(c) Congenital coxa vara

(d) Perthe's disease

Image shows a Pavlik harness.

Answer: A. Developmental dysplasia of the hip

28. A 30 years old male presented with pain and swelling around knee joint. X-ray showed a lesion involving the epiphyseal region of lower end of femur, as shown below. Biopsy of the lesion showed the presence of mononuclear spindle cells and multinucleated giant cells. Most likely diagnosis:

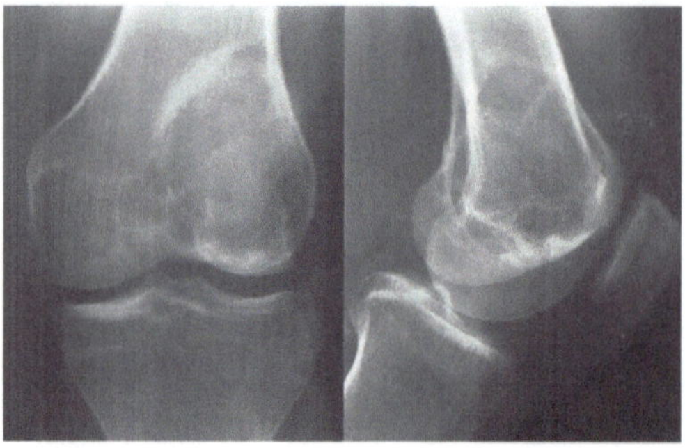

(a) Osteosarcoma (b) Ewing's sarcoma

(c) Osteoid osteoma (d) Osteoclastoma

Answer: D i.e., Osteoclastoma

29. Which of the following is the most common site affected in tuberculosis of hip joint?

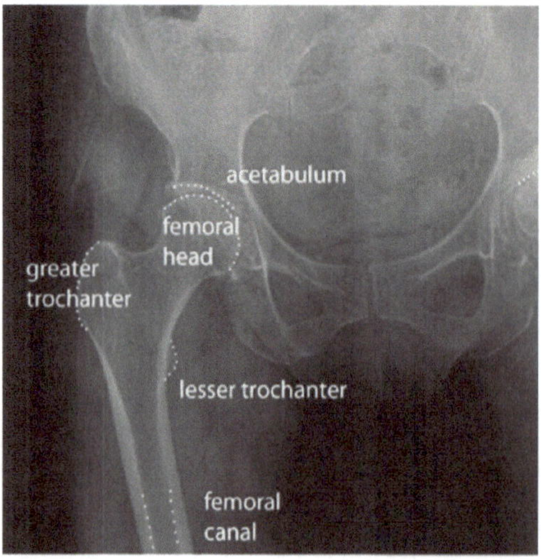

(a) Greater trochanter (b) Femoral head

(c) Acetabulum (d) Lesser trochanter

Answer: C. Acetabulum

30. If the injury shown below in the X-ray is not treated properly, what set of complications would occur:

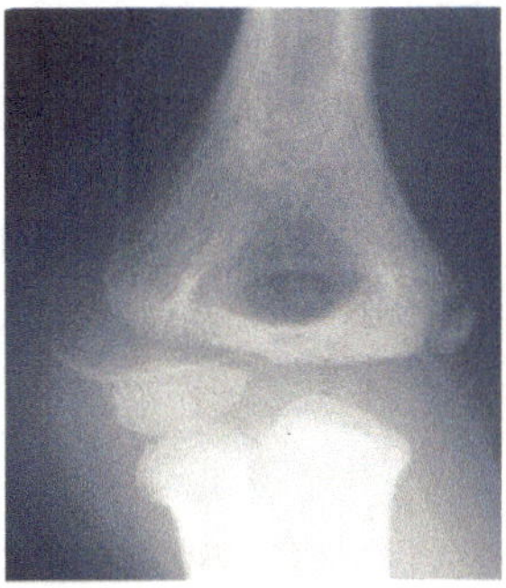

(a) Non-union, Cubitus valgus deformity

(b) Non-union, Cubitus varus deformity

(c) Malunion, Cubitus varus deformity

(d) Malunion, Cubitus valgus deformity

X-shows a displaced lateral condyle fracture of the humerus.

The *lateral condyle fracture* is a Salter-Harris IV *fracture* pattern and follows physeal injury principles.

If not managed surgically, it can go into non-union and consequent cubitus valgus deformity.

Answer: A i.e., Non-union, Cubitus valgus deformity

31. A child presented to the OPD with the complaints of pain in forearm and leg. X-ray showed diaphyseal sclerosis. Peripheral smear of the patient is shown below. Organism responsible for such a problem is:

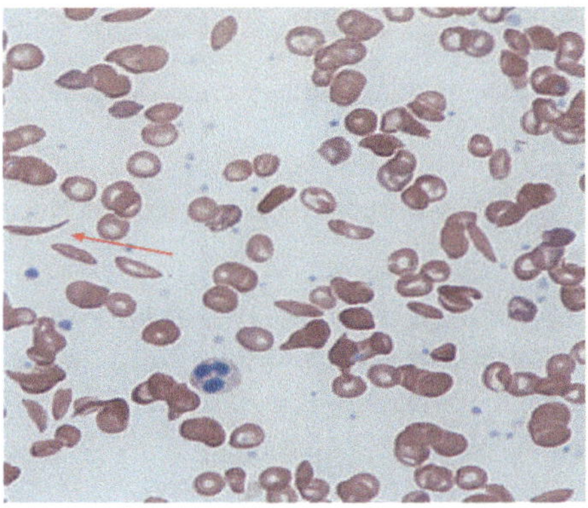

(a) Staphylococcus aureus (b) Salmonella typhii

(c) Streptococcus (d) Mycobacterium TB

Clinical presentation is suggestive of osteomyelitis and peripheral smear is suggestive of sickle cell anemia. *Osteomyelitis* is an infection in a bone. Infections can reach a bone by traveling through the bloodstream or spreading from nearby tissue.

Osteomyelitis in a patient of sickle cell anemia is caused by Salmonella typhii.

Red arrow shows a sickle shaped RBC.

Answer: B i.e., Salmonella typhii

32. **All of the following statements about the condition shown in the image are true EXCEPT:**

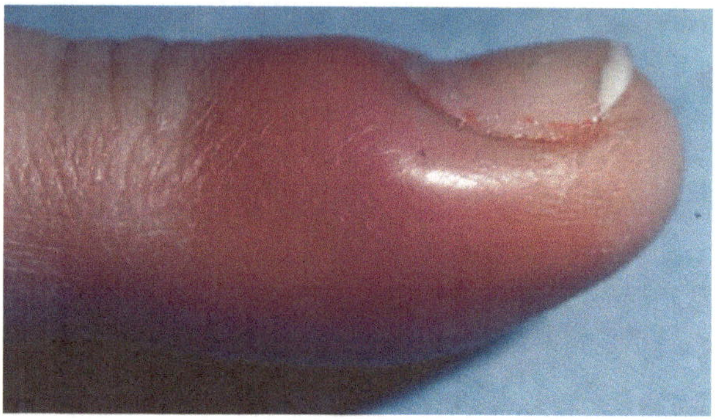

(a) Most commonly caused by staphylococcus epidermidis

(b) Can be managed by antibiotics initially

(c) May be because of a prick injury

(d) May lead to osteomyelitis

Image shows paronychia and it is commonly caused by staphylococcus aureus.

Answer: A. Most commonly caused by staphylococcus epidermidis

33. **A patient had a blow over the knee joint and presented to the Orthopedic OPD with the complaints of pain and swelling over the knee joint. X-ray was done as shown below. Best management for the fracture show in the image:**

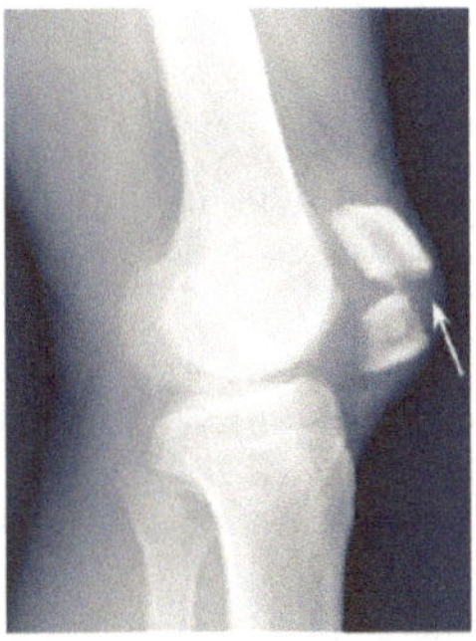

(a) Partial patellectomy

(b) Total patellectomy

(c) Plaster of Paris cast application

(d) Fixation with K-wires and stainless steel/ SS wires

Image shows a displaced two-part fracture of patella, which is best managed by tension band wiring (TBW).

TBW uses K-wires and SS wires.

Patella Fractures are traumatic knee injuries caused by direct trauma or rapid contracture of the quadriceps with a flexed knee.

Answer: D i.e., Fixation with K-wires and stainless steel/ SS wires

34. A young female presented with the complaints of back pain and deformity. She is also having a history of fever and weight loss. Local examination revealed a kyphotic deformity. Tenderness was elicited on palpation. Movements were restricted. Treating doctor advised for MRI scan as shown below. Most likely diagnosis:

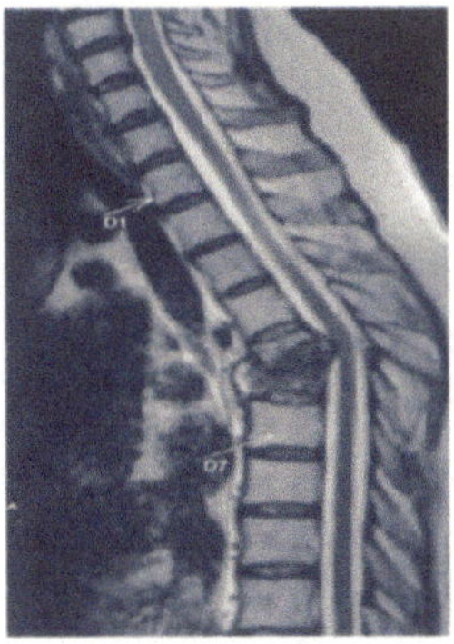

(a) Metastasis to spine (b) Ankylosing spondylitis

(c) Spondylolisthesis (d) Tuberculosis of the spine

Clinical presentation and image are indicative of TB spine.

Spinal tuberculosis causes the destruction, collapse of vertebrae, and angulation of vertebral column. The progression of spinal tuberculosis is slow and insidious. The total duration of the illness varies from few months to few years, with average disease duration ranging from 4 to 11 months.

MRI of the spine is the investigation of choice to evaluate the type and extent of compression of spinal cord in TB spine. It also shows the condition of the underlying neural tissues, and thus helps in predicting the prognosis.

Answer: D i.e., Tuberculosis of the spine

35. A patient met with Road Traffic Accident and had fracture of the shaft of humerus. After injury, he was unable to dorsiflex the wrist. Orthopedic surgeon advised him a splint as shown in the figure. Identify the splint:

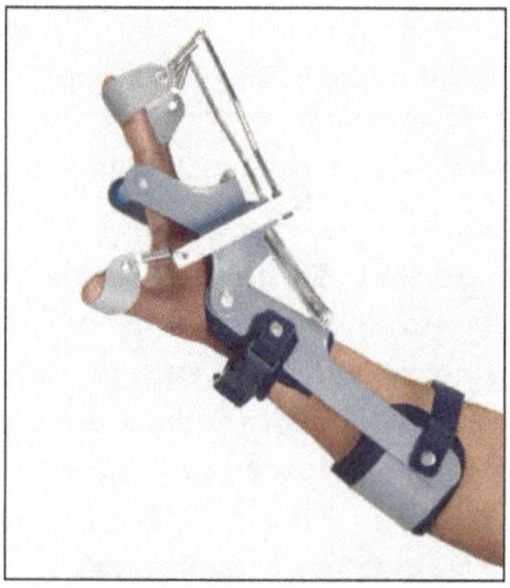

(a) Static cock-up splint (b) Dynamic cock-up splint

(c) Knuckle bender splint (d) Aeroplane splint

Clinical presentation and image are indicative of radial nerve palsy.

Image shows a dynamic cock-up splint.

Fracture shaft of the humerus can cause radial nerve palsy, which manifest as wrist drop. In case of radial nerve palsy, cock-up splint is used.

Answer: B i.e., Dynamic cock-up splint

36. A young male presented with vague pain and swelling around the wrist joint. Imaging studies are shown below. Most likely diagnosis:

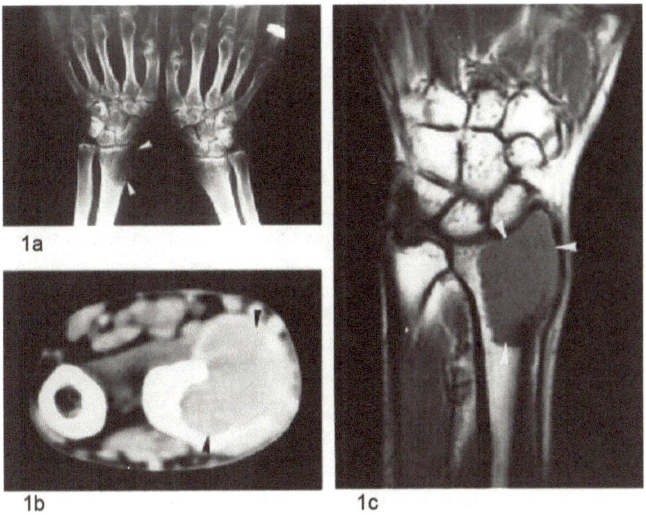

(a) Giant cell tumour
(b) Osteosarcoma
(c) Ewing's sarcoma
(d) Multiple myeloma

Clinical presentation and image are indicative of giant cell tumour.

X-ray shows soap-bubble appearance suggestive of osteoclastoma/ giant cell tumour.

Answer: A i.e., Giant cell tumour

37. A person sitting in the front seat of the car met with a Road Traffic Accident. Following injury, his right lower limb was in flexion, adduction and internal rotation. X-ray of the pelvis with the hips was done as shown below. Most likely diagnosis:

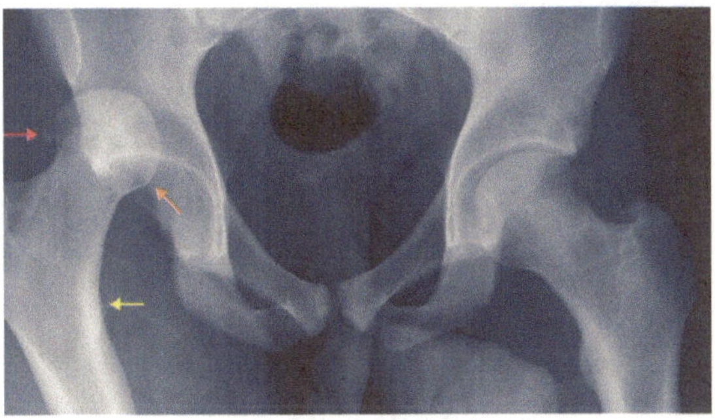

(a) Anterior dislocation of the hip
(b) Posterior dislocation of the hip
(c) Fracture neck of femur
(d) Fracture subtrochanter femur

Clinical presentation and image are indicative of posterior dislocation of right hip.

In approximately 90% of hip dislocation patients, the femur is pushed out of the socket in a backward direction. This is called a posterior dislocation. A posterior dislocation leaves the lower leg in a fixed position, with the knee and foot rotated in toward the middle of the body.

Flexion, **AD**duction and **I**nternal **R**otation (FADIR) attitude suggest posterior dislocation of the limb.

Answer: B i.e., Posterior dislocation of the hip

38. An elderly male presented with multiple bony pain, anemia, renal failure, proteinuria and hypercalcemia. X-ray skull was done as shown below. Most likely diagnosis:

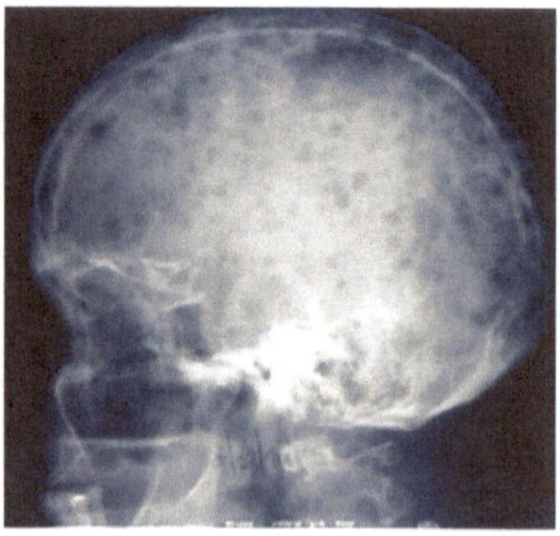

(a) Multiple myeloma
(b) Metastasis to skull
(c) Primary hyperparathyroidism
(d) Secondary hyperparathyroidism

Clinical presentation and image are indicative of multiple myeloma.

Multiple myeloma is a type of cancer that occurs when an atypical plasma cell develops in the bone marrow and reproduces quickly.

X-ray shows multiple punched out lesion, very suggestive of multiple myeloma.

Answer: A i.e., Multiple myeloma

39. A 30 years old male presented with vague pain and swelling in wrist region. X-ray showed a lytic lesion which eroded the cortex of the bone. Histopathological image of the lesion is shown below. Most likely diagnosis:

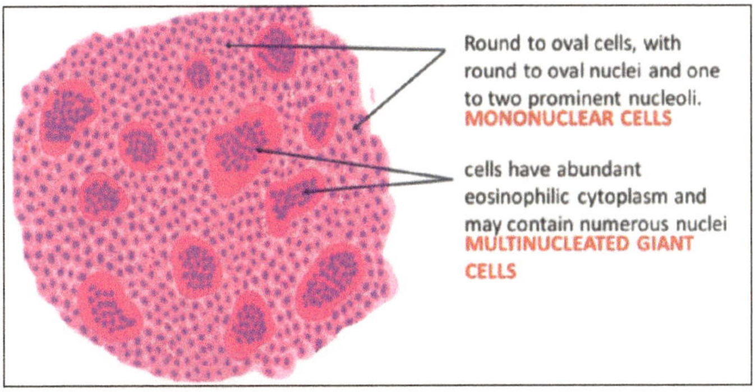

(a) Giant cell tumour (b) Osteosarcoma
(c) Ewing's sarcoma (d) Osteochondroma

Clinical history and histopathological image are indicative of giant cell tumour.

The giant cell tumor of bone (GCTB), also known as an osteoclastoma or a myeloid sarcoma, is a benign local aggressive osteolytic neoplasm that primarily affects skeletally mature young adults.

Histopathology shows multinucleated giant cells and mononuclear spindle cells.

Answer: A i.e., Giant cell tumour

40. A patient from Bihar presented to the OPD with some bone and teeth problems. Clinical image of the teeths and X-ray of forearm is shown below. Most likely diagnosis:

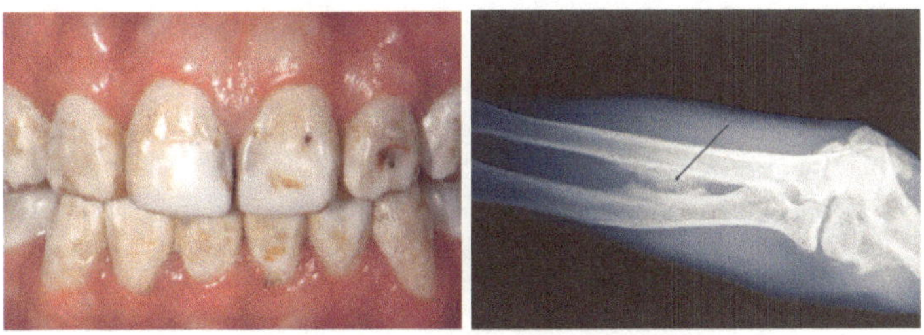

(a) Fluorosis (b) Osteoporosis
(c) Dental caries (d) Osteosclerosis

Clinical presentation and images are indicative of fluorosis.

Fluorosis is a crippling disease resulted from deposition of fluorides in the hard and soft tissues of body.

Dental fluorosis is the earliest sign of fluorosis. The earliest to occur is mottling of the enamel, best seen in the incisors of the upper jaw. There may be interosseous membrane calcification in forearm (shown with black arrow) and leg.

Answer: A i.e., Fluorosis

41. A 25 years old male presented with vague pain and swelling around the wrist joints since last 4 months. Clinical image and the X-ray are shown below. Most likely diagnosis:

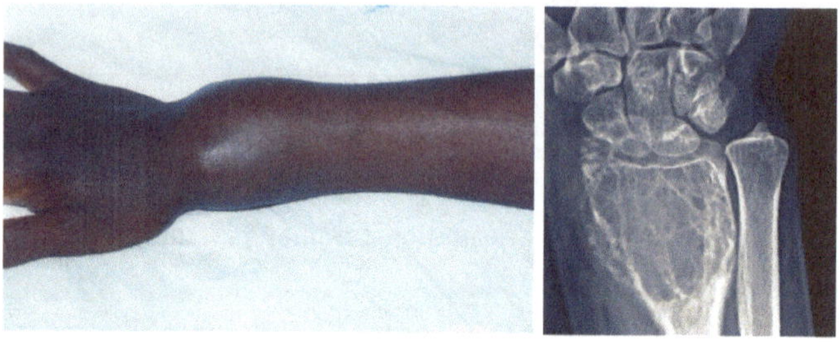

(a) Osteosarcoma (b) Ewing's sarcoma

(c) Giant cell tumour (d) Enchondroma

Clinical presentation and images are indicative of giant cell tumour.

Giant cell tumors (GCTs) of bone, also known as *osteoclastomas*, are benign locally lytic bone lesions that occur most commonly in men aged 20–40 years of age.

X-ray shows soap bubble appearance.

Answer: C i.e., Giant cell tumour

42. Which nerve is being checked by the clinical test shown in the image:

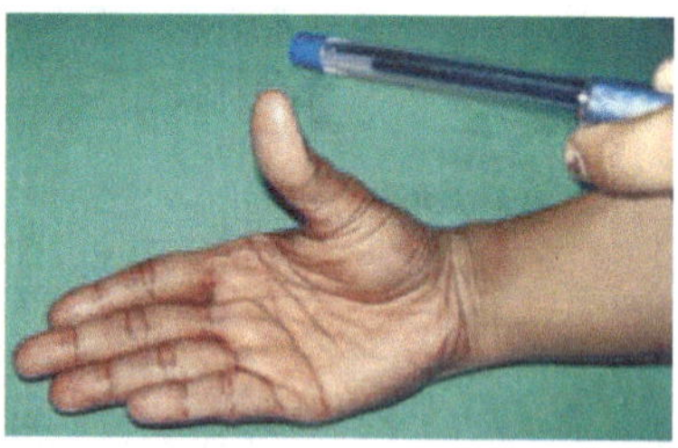

(a) Median nerve (b) Radial nerve

(c) Ulnar nerve (d) Axillary nerve

Clinical test performed is a pen test.

Pen test checks median nerve.

Positive *pen test* (paralysis of abductor pollicis brevis) – unable to touch the object held above the thumb at right angle to the thumb.

Answer: A i.e., Median nerve

43. Age group commonly affected in the condition shown below:

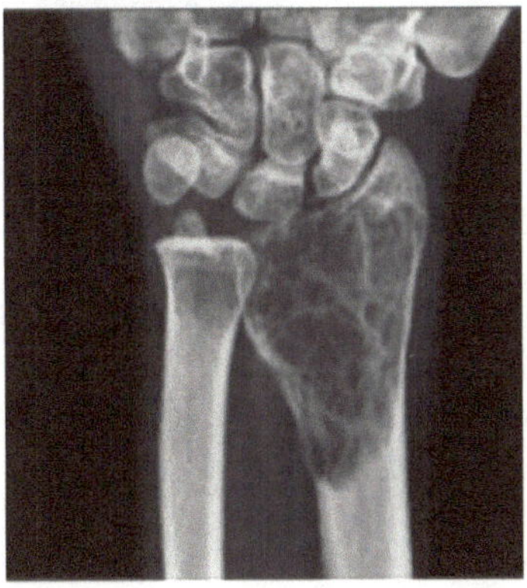

(a) 10-20 years (b) 20-40 years

(c) 40-60 years (d) 60-80 years

Giant cell tumour is commonly seen in 20-40 years of age.

Answer: B i.e., 20-40 years

44. Radiological feature shown in the image below is:

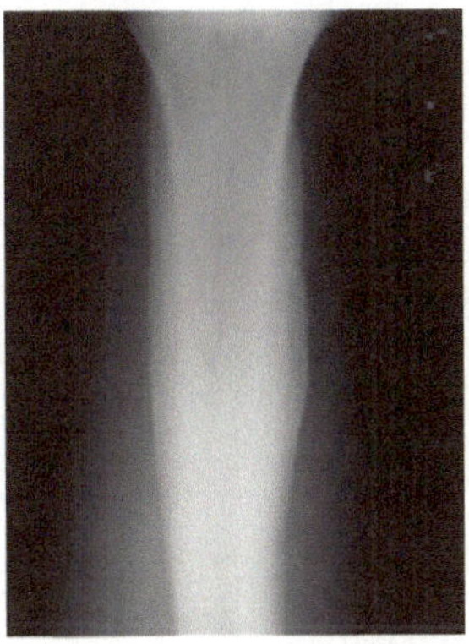

(a) Soap bubble appearance (b) Codman's triangle

(c) Onion peel appearance (d) Sun-ray appearance

In a typical case of Ewing's sarcoma, there is a lytic lesion in the medullary zone of the midshaft of a long bone, with cortical destruction and new bone formation in layers – onion peel appearance.

Answer: C i.e., Onion peel appearance

45. Management of the fracture shown below:

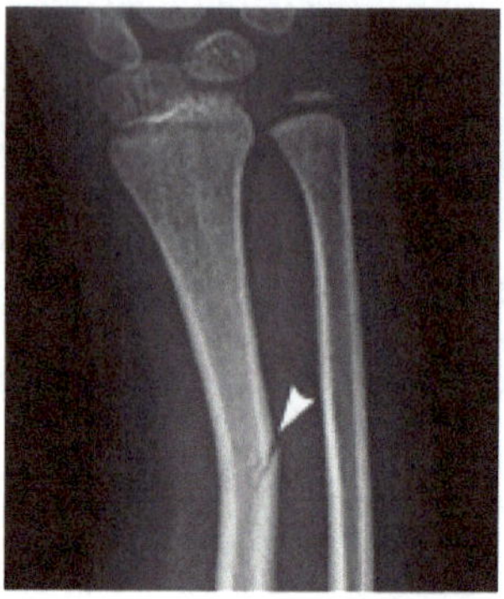

(a) Closed reduction (b) Open reduction

(c) Internal fixation (d) Observation

Greenstick fractures are managed by closed reduction by manipulation under general anesthesia (after completing the fracture line), and immobilization in an above-elbow plaster cast.

Answer: A i.e., Closed reduction

46. Management of the fracture shown below:

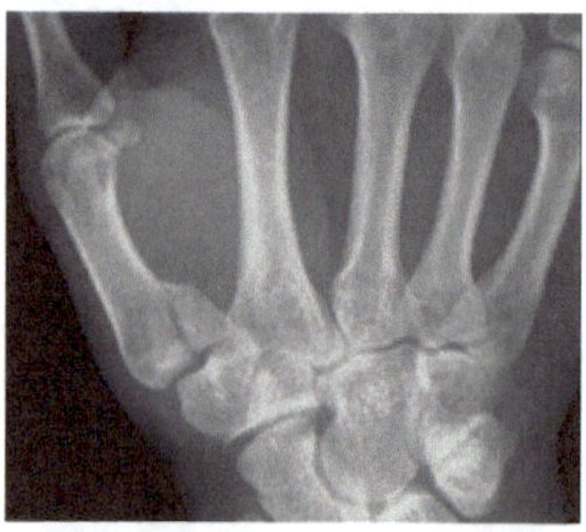

(a) Closed reduction & cast

(b) Closed reduction & fixation

(c) Observation

(d) Excision of trapezium

Bennet's fracture-dislocation needs accurate reduction and restoration of the smooth joint surface. This is because, being an intra-articular fracture, if not reduced accurately, it will lead to incongruity of the articular surfaces. This would increase the chances of developing osteoarthritis. This can be done by closed reduction/ open reduction with K-wire fixation.

Answer: B i.e., Closed reduction and fixation

47. Such splint is used in which nerve injury:

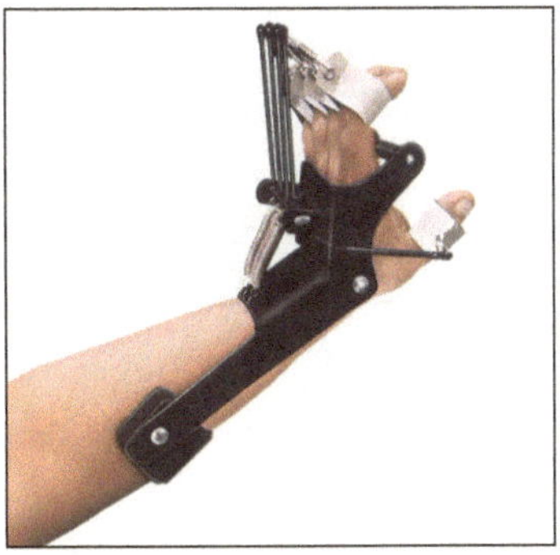

(a) Ulnar nerve
(b) Median nerve
(c) Radial nerve
(d) Axillary nerve

Cock-up splint is used for radial nerve palsy.

Answer: C i.e., Radial nerve

48. Splint shown is used for which condition:

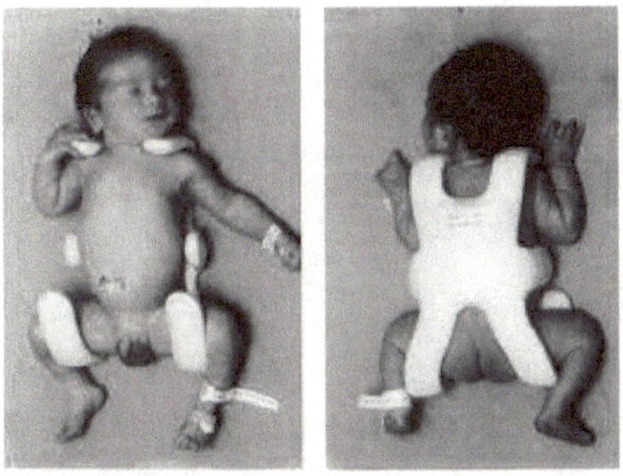

(a) Fracture neck of femur

(b) Developmental dysplasia of hip

(c) Perthe's disease

(d) Coxa vara

While managing DDH, once the hip has been reduced by closed or open methods, Von Rosen's splint is used for maintaining the head of femur inside the acetabulum. It can be removed once the acetabulum develops to a round shape.

Answer: B i.e., Developmental dysplasia of hip

49. Which nerve is injured?

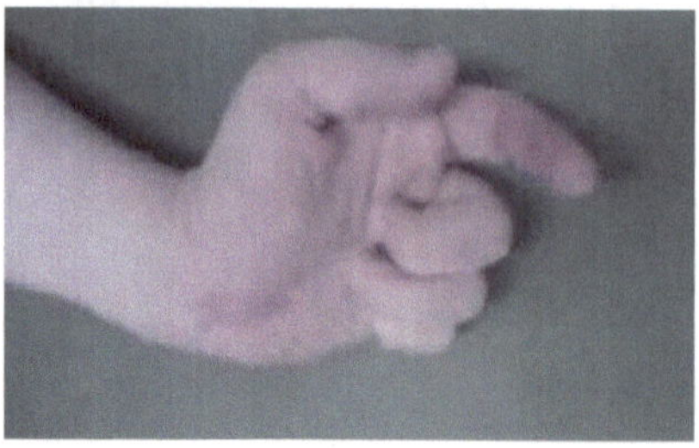

(a) Median nerve (b) Ulnar nerve

(c) Radial nerve (d) Axillary nerve

On asking the patient to make a fist, it is noticed that the index finger remains straight (pointing index). This is due to paralysis of both the flexors (digitorum superficialis and lateral half of the digitorum profundus) of the index finger, which occurs in median nerve palsy at the level proximal to the elbow. The other fingers can be flexed by functioning medial side of the flexor digitorum profundus, supplied by the ulnar nerve.

Answer: A i.e., Median nerve

50. X-ray is suggestive of:

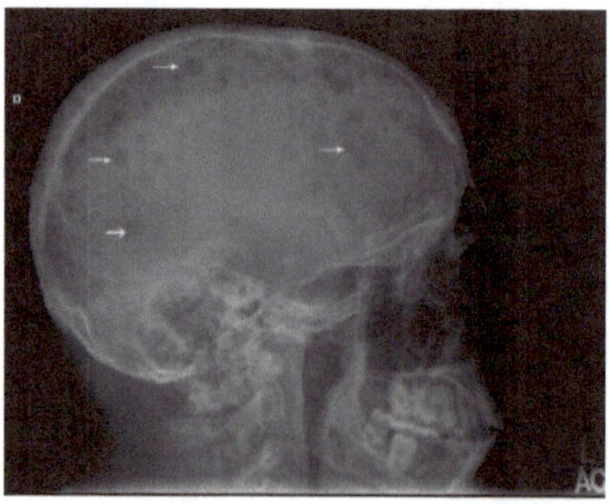

(a) Thalassemia (b) Sickle cell anemia

(c) Multiple myeloma (d) Secondaries

Multiple punched out lesions in the skull and other flat bones is suggestive of multiple myeloma.

Answer: C i.e., Multiple myeloma

51. A child presented with pain in the forearm following a trauma. An AP and lateral X-ray of the forearm revealed the findings as shown in the X-ray. Most likely diagnosis:

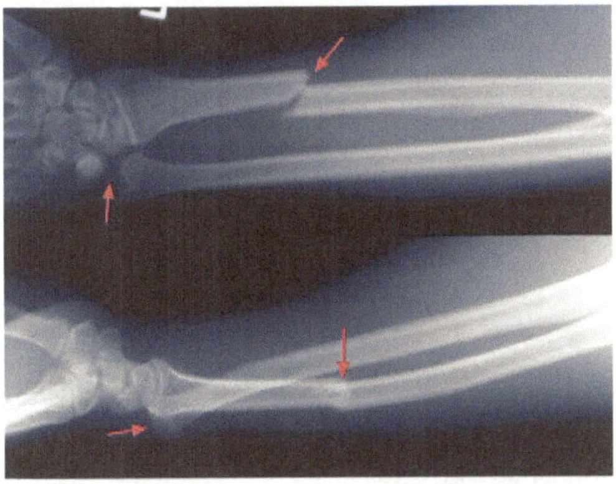

(a) Monteggia fracture (b) Colle's fracture

(c) Smith's fracture (d) Galeazzi's fracture

X-ray shows fracture of lower third of radius and there is dislocation of inferior radio-ulnar joint

Answer: D i.e., Galeazzi's fracture

52. Eponym for the type of fracture shown below:

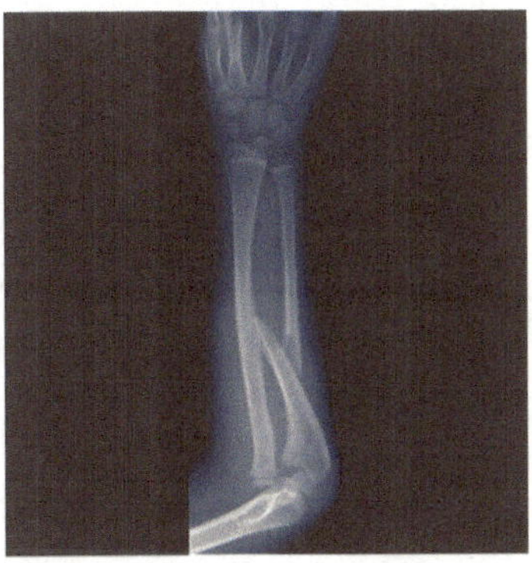

(a) Galeazzi fracture dislocation

(b) Monteggia fracture dislocation

(c) Colle's fracture

(d) Smith's fracture

X-ray shows fracture of proximal third of ulna and dislocation of superior radio-ulnar joint.

Answer: B i.e., Monteggia fracture dislocation

53. Identify the prosthesis:

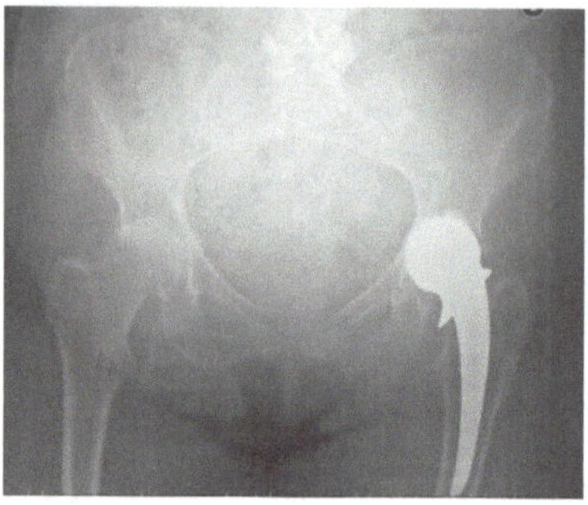

(a) Austin Moore prosthesis

(b) Thompson prosthesis

(c) Bipolar prosthesis

(d) Total hip replacement prosthesis

Thompson prosthesis is used in hemi-replacement arthroplasty of hip (replacement of femoral head), following fracture neck of femur in elderly.

Answer: B i.e., Thompson prosthesis

54. Identify the deformity shown in the image:

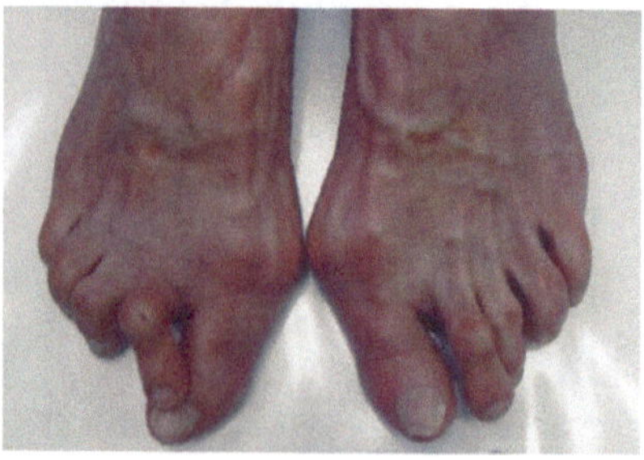

(a) Hallux varus (b) Hallux valgus

(c) Pes planus (d) Pes cavus

Hallux valgus is the lateral deviation of the great toe at the metatarso-phalangeal joint.

Answer: B i.e., Hallux valgus

55. The following pelvic X-ray was seen in a patient. All of the following clinical test/ signs are associated with this condition EXCEPT:

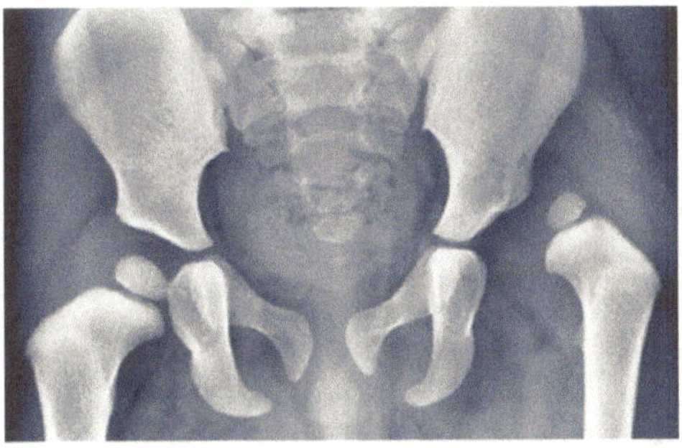

(a) Ortolani (b) Barlow

(c) Narath (d) Gaenslen

Gaenslen test is done for sacro-ilitis.

Answer: D i.e., Gaenslen

56. Identify the clinical sign shown in the image:

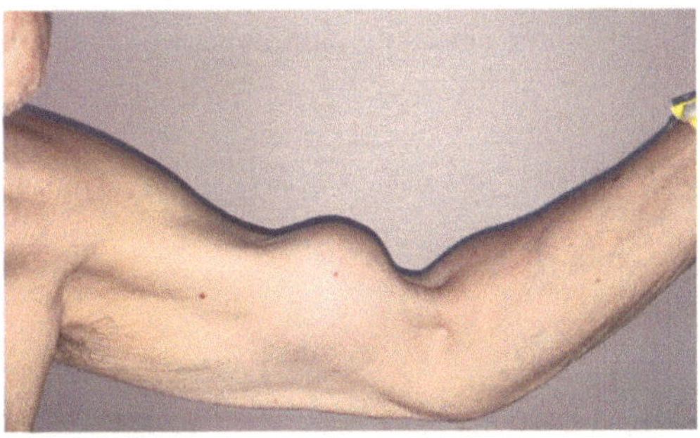

(a) Popeye sign (b) Trenthovan sign

(c) Aneurysmal sign (d) Regimental badge sign

Image shows Popeye sign.

Popeye sign is seen in rupture of long head of biceps brachii muscle

A degenerate tendon can rupture causing the muscle to retract down the arm. This can alter the contour of your biceps to give a 'Popeye Sign'.

Answer: A i.e., Popeye sign

57. **A 30 years old male presented with pain and swelling around knee joint. Biopsy of the lesion showed the presence of mononuclear spindle cells and multinucleated giant cells, as shown in the image below. Most likely diagnosis:**

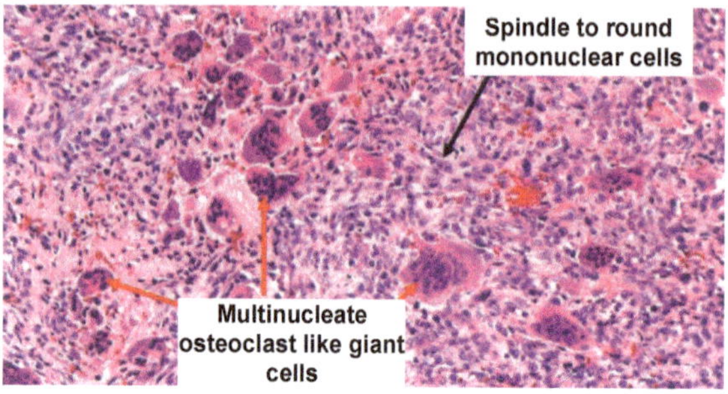

(a) Osteosarcoma (b) Ewing's sarcoma
(c) Osteoid osteoma (d) Osteoclastoma

Histopathological image shows feature of giant cell tumour.

Giant cell tumor (GCT) of bone is generally a benign tumor composed of mononuclear stromal cells and characteristic multi-nucleated giant cells.

Histopathology of giant cell tumour shows the presence of mononuclear spindle cells and multinucleated giant cells.

Answer: D i.e., Osteoclastoma

58. **Identify the clinical test shown below:**

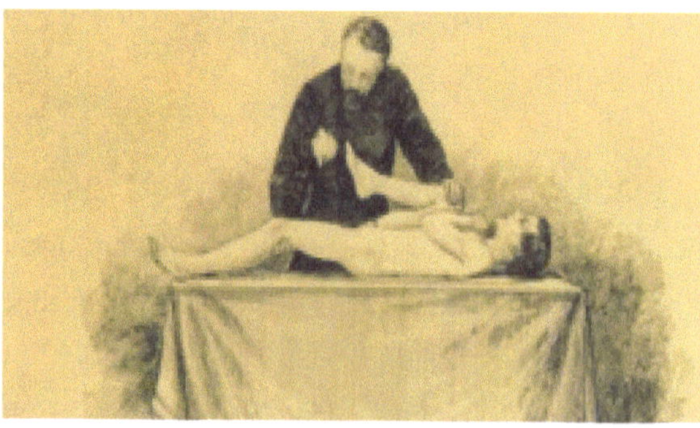

(a) Straight leg raising test (b) Sign of Narath

(c) Thomas test (d) Trendelenburg test

Thomas test checks the fixed flexion deformity at the hip joint.

Answer: C i.e., Thomas test

59. A 30 years old male presented with hip pain for the last 6 months. X-ray of the hip is shown below. Most likely diagnosis:

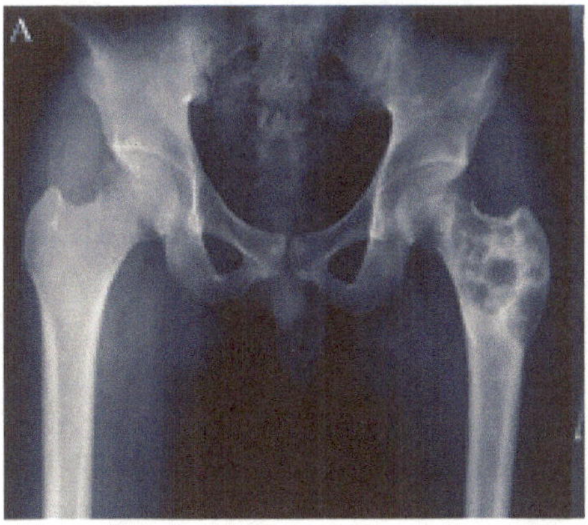

(a) Giant cell tumour (b) Simple bone cyst

(c) Adamantinoma (d) Ewing's sarcoma

Soap bubble appearance is suggestive of giant cell tumour.

Answer: A i.e., Giant cell tumour

60. Identify the condition shown below:

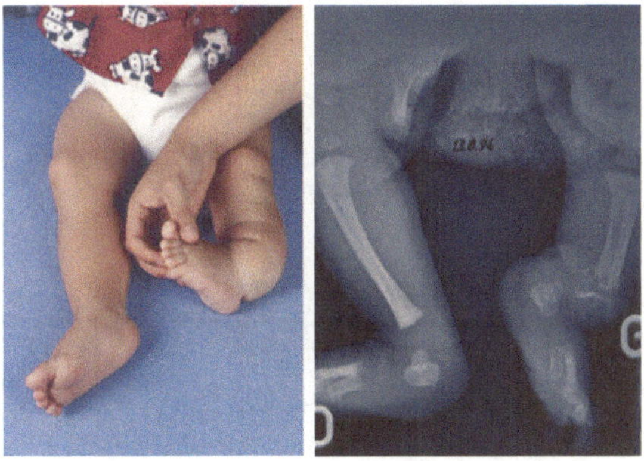

(a) Tibial hemimelia

(b) Fibular hemimelia

(c) Congenital pseudo-arthrosis of tibia

(d) Tibial torsion

Congenital pseudo-arthrosis of tibia is characterized by segmental osseous weakness, resulting in anterolateral angulation of the tibia. The osseous dysplasia leads to a tibial non-union, because of tibial bowing and reduced growth in the distal tibial epiphysis, shortening of the limb occurs.

Answer: C i.e., Congenital pseudo-arthrosis of tibia

61. A 30 years young lady presented with the complaints of pain and stiffness in multiple joints of the hand, particularly in the morning. Hand shows the deformity as shown in the image below. Most likely diagnosis:

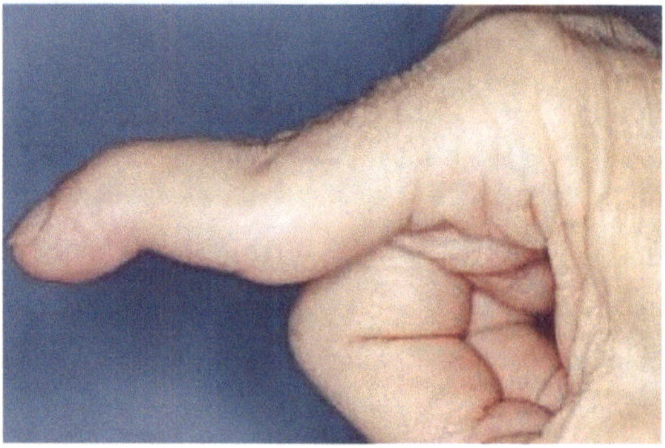

(a) Osteoarthritis (b) Rheumatoid arthritis

(c) Psoriatic arthritis (d) SLE

Clinical presentation and image are indicative of rheumatoid arthritis.

RA is a chronic disease that causes joint pain, stiffness, swelling and decreased movement of the joints. Small joints in the hands and feet are most commonly affected.

Image shows a typical swan-neck deformity

Answer: B i.e., Rheumatoid arthritis

62. A 60 years old post-menopausal lady presented with the complaints of low back pain. X-ray of the spine was done which is shown below. Most likely diagnosis:

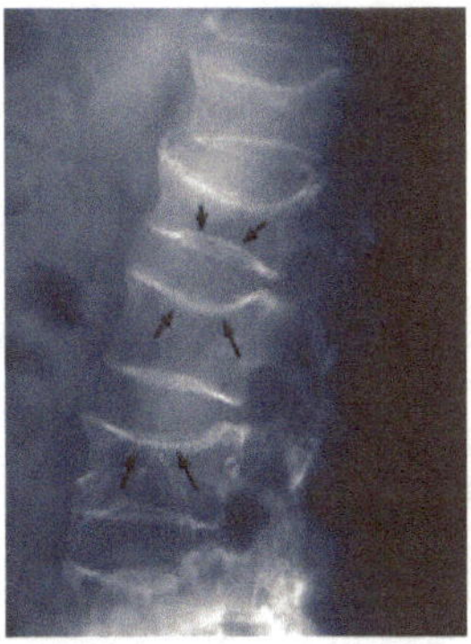

(a) Rheumatoid arthritis (b) Osteoarthritis

(c) Osteopetrosis (d) Osteoporosis

X-ray shows osteoporosis.

Osteoporosis is a bone disease that develops when bone mineral density and bone mass decreases.

X-ray features include cod-fish appearance in which the disc bulges into the adjacent vertebral bodies so that the disc becomes biconvex (black arrows).

Answer: D i.e., Osteoporosis

63. A child had a fall on ground over his left shoulder. After this, he presented to the Orthopedic OPD with the complaints of pain and swelling over left shoulder and he was supporting his left elbow with right hand. X-ray of the child is shown below. Which of the bone is fractured:

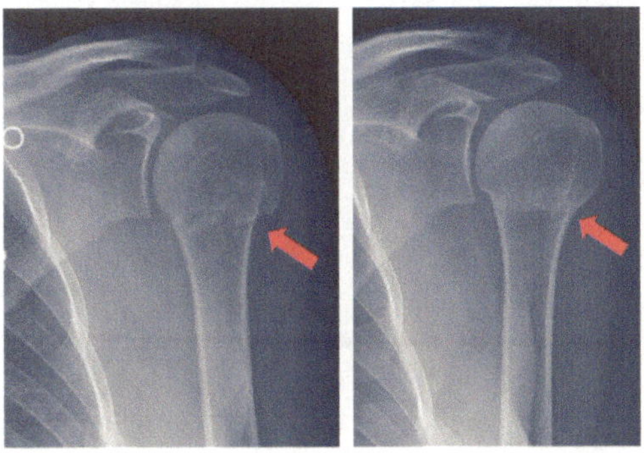

(a) Clavicle (b) Scapula

(c) Ribs (d) Humerus

X-ray shows fracture of proximal humerus.

Proximal humeral fractures usually result from a fall on an outstretched arm.

Answer: D i.e., Humerus

64. In the given case, calculation of the deformity is done by measuring:

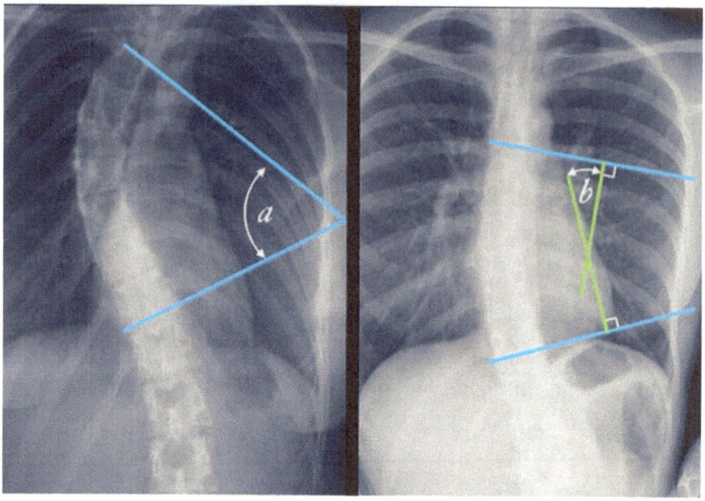

(a) Kite's angle (b) Cobb's angle

(c) Q angle (d) Bryant's angle

X-ray is indicative of scoliosis and Cobb's angle is measured.

Scoliosis is a sideways curvature of the spine. Scoliosis is a sideways curvature of the spine that most often is diagnosed in adolescents.

For proper assessment of scoliosis, a full antero-posterior X-ray of the spine in supine and erect position, plus a lateral view are necessary. Severity of the curve is measured by Cobb's angle - an angle between the line passing through the margins of the vertebrae at the ends of the curve.

Answer: B i.e., Cobb's angle

CLINICAL MCQs

1. A young patient presented to the Orthopedic OPD with pain and swelling around the shoulder joint after a fall on outstretched hand. After thorough clinical examination, treating doctor suspected it to be a case of fracture clavicle. What is the most common site of fracture clavicle?

(a) Junction of lateral half and medial half

(b) Junction of medial one-third and lateral two-third

(c) Junction of medial two-third and lateral one-third

(d) Medial half

The clavicle (collarbone) is one of the most fractured bones in the body.

Most common site of fracture clavicle is junction of medial 2/3rd and lateral 1/3rd.

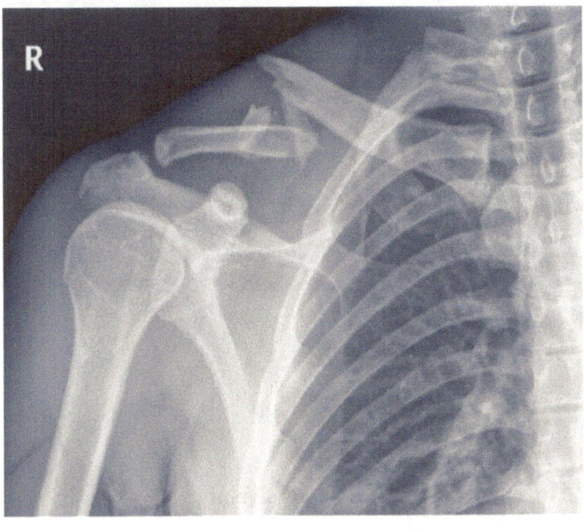

Answer: C i.e., Junction of medial two-third and lateral one-third

2. A patient was operated on hand for some pathology, but after the surgery, he was not able to flex the index finger. Which structure is most probably damaged:

(a) Median nerve (b) Ulnar nerve

(c) Radial nerve (d) Flexor pollicis longus

Clinical presentation is suggestive of median nerve palsy.

The deformity discussed is pointing index.

"*Pointing* finger" deformity is caused due to injury to the median nerve in the mid-forearm by paralysis of flexor digitorum superficialis.

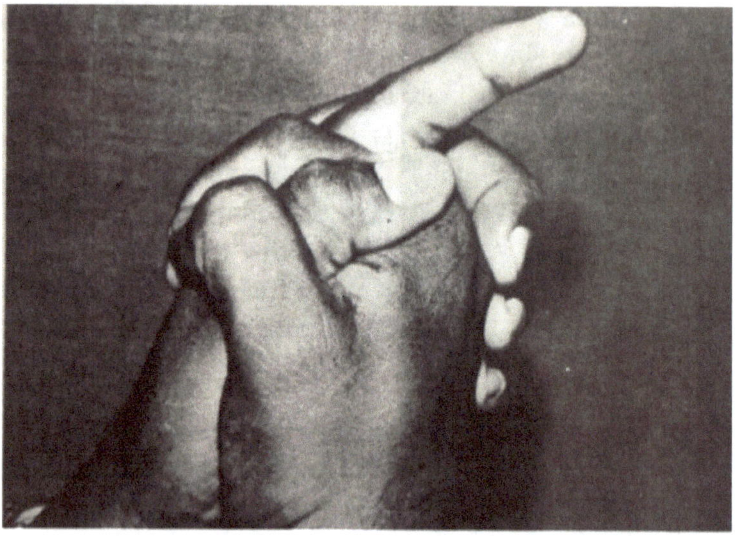

Answer: A i.e., Median nerve

3. A young male had pain in the right hip joint since few months. He was examined by an Orthopedic surgeon and it was found that there is true shortening of the right lower limb. There is no history of trauma. Most likely diagnosis:

(a) Stage of synovitis of TB hip

(b) Stage of the arthritis of TB hip

(c) Stage of erosion of TB hip

(d) Avascular necrosis of head of femur

After the spine, the *hip* joint is the most common site of involvement for *tuberculosis, and* constitutes approximately 15% of all cases.

Staging	Clinical findings	Radiologic features
I. Stage of synovitis	Flexion, abduction, external rotation, apparent lengthening	Haziness, rarefaction
II. Stage of early arthritis	Flexion, adduction, internal rotation, apparent shortening	Rarefaction, osteopenia, bony lesion in femoral head, acetabulum or both. No reduction in joint space
III. Stage of arthritis	Flexion, adduction, internal rotation, shortening	All of the above and destruction of articular surface, reduction in joint space
IV. Stage of advanced arthritis	Flexion, adduction, internal rotation with gross shortening	Complete destruction, no joint space, wandering acetabulum

Answer: C i.e., Stage of erosion of TB hip

4. **An alcoholic patient slept at the night keeping his head over the arm. Next morning, when he woke up, his radial nerve was paralysed. This is which kind of injury:**

(a) Neurapraxia (b) Axonotmesis

(c) Neurotmesis (d) Wallerian degeneration

Neurapraxia is a mild form of nerve damage that can lead to temporary motor and sensory loss. *Neurapraxia* is the mildest form of peripheral nerve injury.

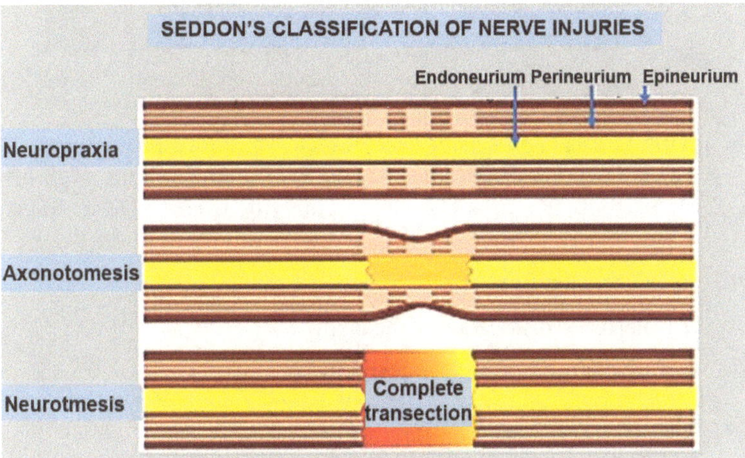

Answer: A i.e., Neurapraxia

5. **A 24 years old male, a known epileptic, presented to following a seizure with pain in the right shoulder region. Examination revealed that the right upper limb was adducted and externally rotated and the movements could not be performed. Most likely diagnosis:**

   (a) Luxatio erecta

   (b) Posterior dislocation of the shoulder

   (c) Intra-thoracic dislocation of the shoulder

   (d) Subglenoid dislocation of the shoulder

   Clinical presentation is suggestive of posterior dislocation of the shoulder

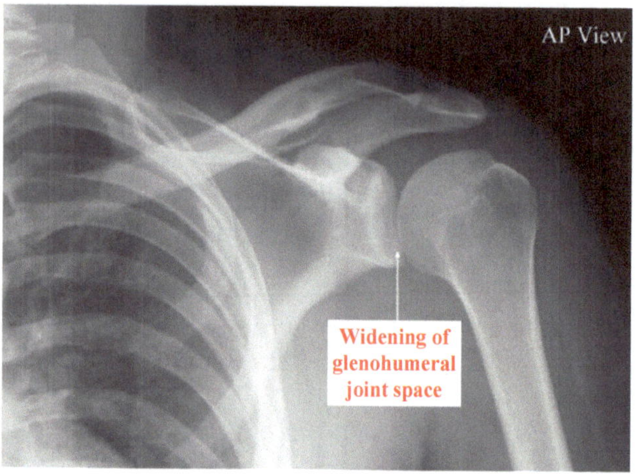

Answer: B i.e., Posterior dislocation of the shoulder

6. **After falling from a height, a child lands on his fully outstretched hands. On examination, there is pain and swelling over his right elbow. There is S-shaped deformity at elbow. Most likely diagnosis:**

   (a) Olecranon fracture

   (b) Posterior dislocation of the elbow

   (c) Fracture supracondylar humerus

   (d) Fracture both bone forearm

   Clinical presentation is suggestive of fracture supracondylar humerus

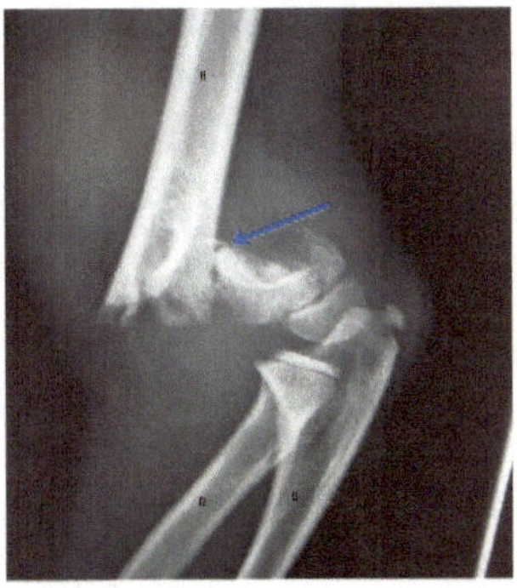

Answer: C i.e., Fracture supracondylar humerus

7. **Q. A 10 years old boy presenting with a cubitus varus deformity and a history of trauma 3 months back. On examination, the three point-bony relationship is preserved. Most likely diagnosis:**

   (a) Old unreduced dislocation of elbow

   (b) Non-union of lateral humeral condylar fracture

   (c) Malunited inter-condylar fracture of the humerus

   (d) Malunited supracondylar fracture of the humerus

   Clinical presentation is suggestive of malunited supracondylar fracture of the humerus

   Supracondylar fracture malunion usually results in cubitus varus deformity.

   3-points bony relationship is maintained as the fracture line is above the landmarks (line joining medial epicondyle and lateral epicondyle).

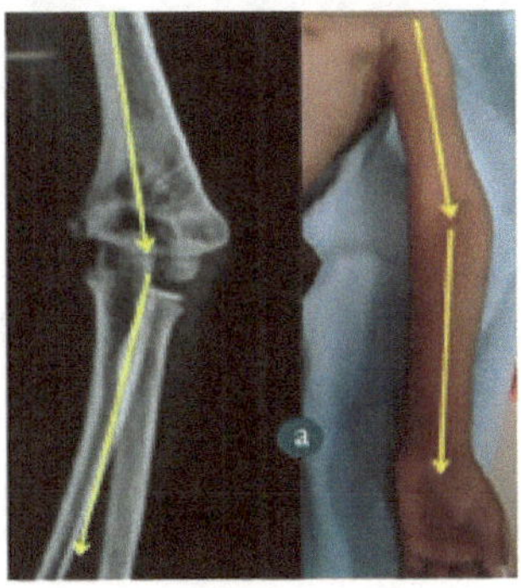

Answer: D i.e., Malunited supracondylar fracture of the humerus

8. A patient sustained injury to the upper limb 3 years back; he now presents with valgus deformity in the elbow and paresthesia over the medial border of the hand. Most likely diagnosis:

(a) Supracondylar humerus fracture

(b) Lateral condyle humerus fracture

(c) Medial condyle humerus fracture

(d) Posterior dislocation of elbow

Clinical presentation is suggestive of old lateral condylar fracture, which has failed to unite, resulting in cubitus valgus deformity and features of ulnar nerve involvement (paresthesia over medial border of the hand).

Therefore operative fixation of a displaced fracture lateral humeral condyle is a must.

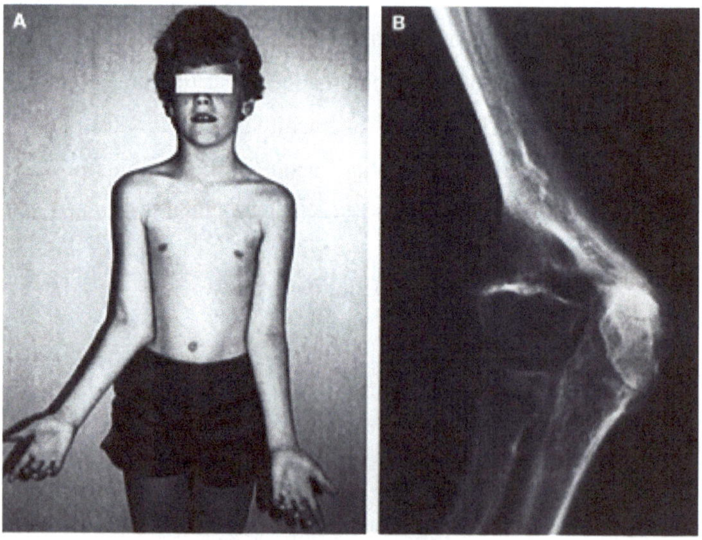

Answer: B i.e., Lateral condyle humerus fracture

9. A child is spinned around, by his father holding the hand. Suddenly, the child started crying and did not allow his father to touch the elbow. Most likely diagnosis:

(a) Supracondylar fracture of humerus

(b) Pulled elbow

(c) Fracture olecranon process

(d) Radial head fracture

Clinical presentation is suggestive of pulled elbow.

Pulled elbow is defined as a radial head subluxation caused by axial traction or a sudden pull of the extended pronated arm.

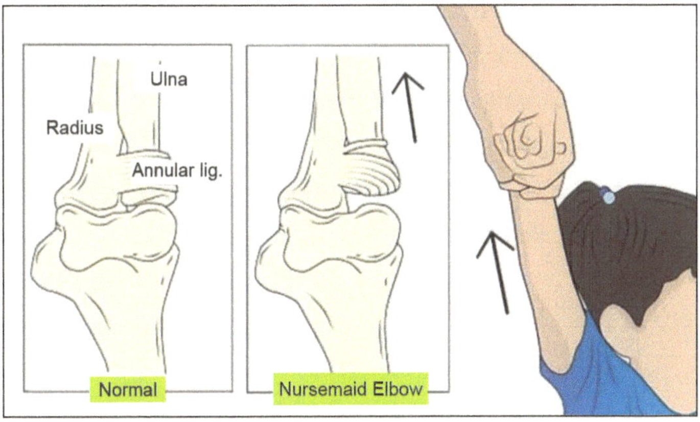

Answer: B i.e., Pulled elbow

10. **3 days after Colle's fracture, a person is not able to extend the thumb. Most likely diagnosis:**

(a) Rupture of EPL tendon (b) Osteoarthritis

(c) Compartment syndrome (d) Shoulder hand syndrome

Clinical presentation is suggestive of rupture of extensor pollicis longus tendon.

Function of EPL is to extend the thumb.

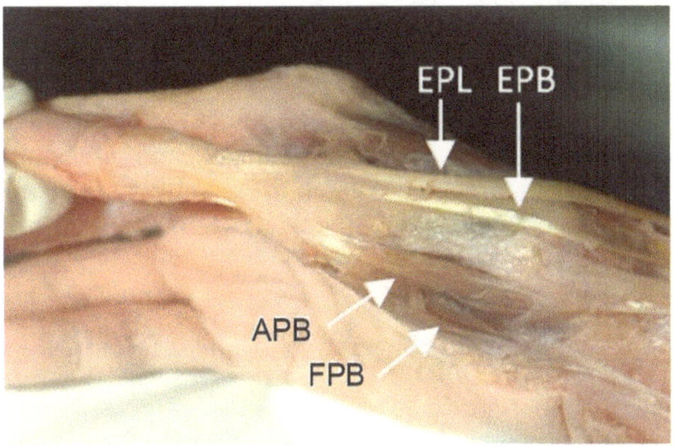

Answer: A i.e., Rupture of Extensor Pollicis Longus tendon

11. A female with Colle's fracture was treated with below elbow cast, presented with severe pain, numbness and paresthesia. Most likely diagnosis:

(a) Unreduced fracture

(b) Compartment syndrome

(c) Reflex sympathetic dystrophy

(d) Malingering

Clinical presentation is suggestive of compartment syndrome.

Acute compartment syndrome is a condition in which there is increased pressure within a closed osteofascial compartment, resulting in ischemia of muscles due to compression of arteries.

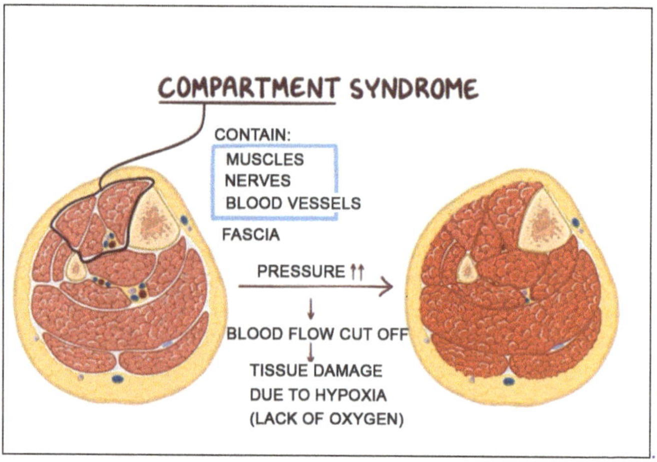

Answer: B i.e., Compartment syndrome

12. Following anterior dislocation of the shoulder, a patient develops weakness of flexion at elbow and lack of sensation over the lateral aspect of forearm. Which nerve is likely to be damaged:

(a) Radial nerve
(b) Musculocutaneous nerve
(c) Axillary nerve
(d) Ulnar nerve

Clinical presentation is suggestive of injury to musculocutaneous nerve.

Flexors of the elbow (biceps and brachialis) are supplied by musculocutaneous nerve.

Sensory nerve supply on the lateral aspect of the forearm is provided by musculocutaneous nerve.

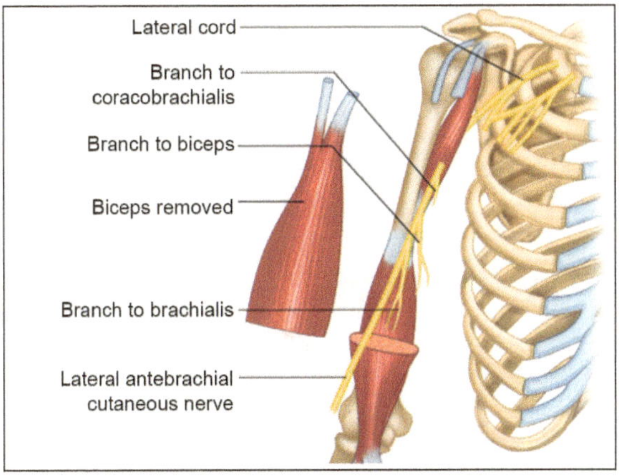

Answer: B i.e., Musculocutaneous nerve

13. **A two years old child was walking holding her father's hand. She suddenly slipped and fell but did not let go her father's hand. After a while, she started crying and was holding the forearm in pronated position. She was afraid of moving the affected extremity. Most appropriate management:**

   (a) Supinate the forearm

   (b) Examine the child under GA

   (c) Elevate the limb and observe

   (d) Investigate for shoulder dislocation

   Clinical presentation is suggestive of pulled elbow.

   It is managed by supination and flexion of the forearm.

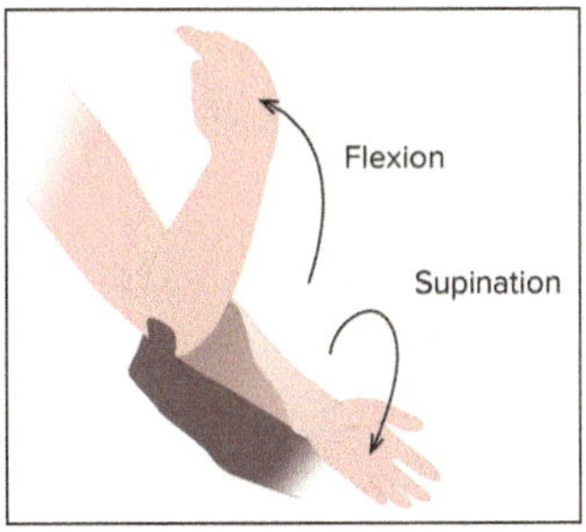

Answer: A i.e., Supinate the forearm

14. **A one and a half years old girl has developed painful elbow after being jerked on the forearm, while lifting by her mother. Next thing to be done in such a case:**

(a) Cuff and collar sling mobilization

(b) Reduction setting and above elbow plaster of Paris cast

(c) X-ray and elevation of the limb in posterior slab

(d) Fully supinate the forearm

Clinical presentation is suggestive of pulled elbow.

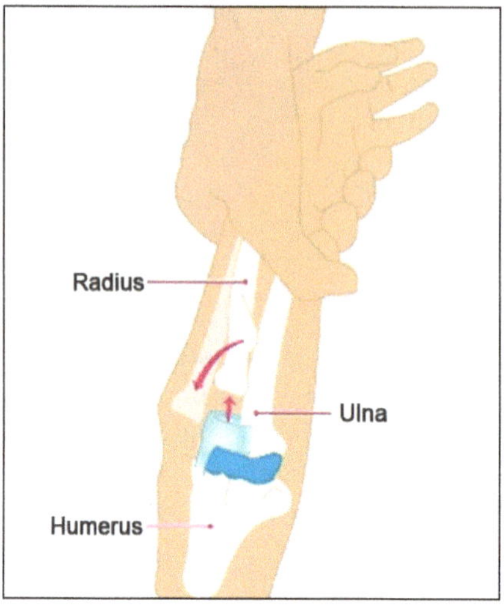

Answer: D i.e., Fully supinate the forearm

15. A 30 years old male involved in a fist-cuff, injured his middle finger and noticed slight flexion of distal interphalangeal joint. X-ray was normal. Most appropriate management:

(a) Ignore

(b) Splint the finger in hyperextension

(c) Surgical repair of the flexor tendon

(d) Buddy strapping

Clinical presentation is suggestive of mallet finger.

A *mallet finger*, also known as hammer finger or PLF finger or Hannan finger, is an extensor tendon injury at the farthest away finger joint.

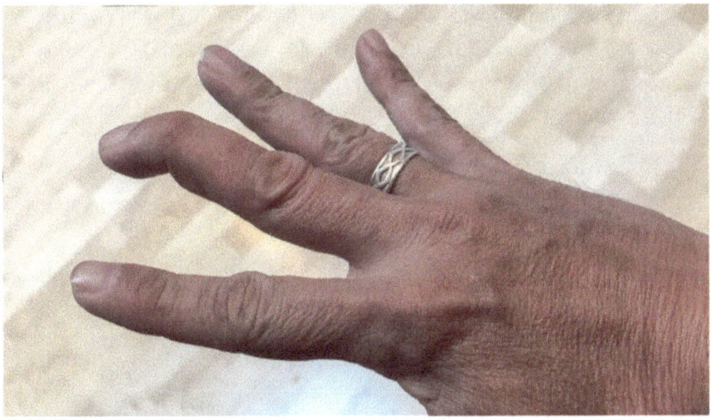

Answer: B i.e., Splint the finger in hyperextension

16. **A 6 years old boy has a history of recurrent dislocation of the right shoulder. During examination, the orthopedician puts the patient in the supine position and abducts his arm to 90 degrees with the bed as the fulcrum and then externally rotates it but the boy does not allow the test to be performed. The test done by the orthopedician is:**

(a) Sulcus test (b) Apprehension test
(c) McMurray's test (d) Apley's test

Patient is scared that his shoulder joint will dislocate again with the maneuver being carried out by the orthopedician. This test is known as apprehension test.

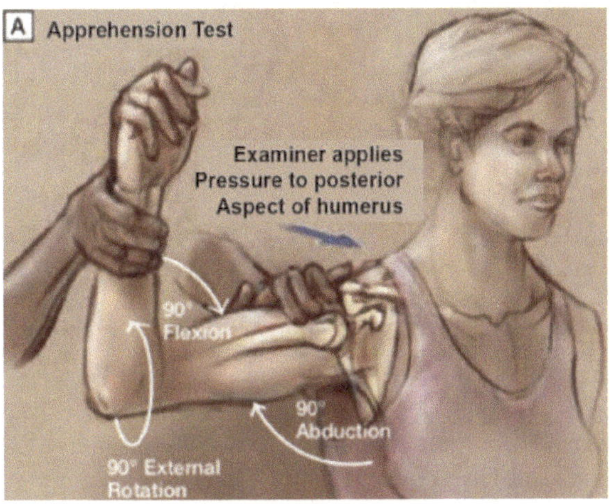

Answer: B i.e., Apprehension test

17. **A 60 years old male fell in the bathroom and was unable to stand. On right hip region, ecchymosis was found. There is external rotation of the leg and the lateral border of foot is touching the bed. Most likely diagnosis:**

(a) Extracapsular fracture neck of femur

(b) Anterior dislocation of the hip

(c) Intracapsular fracture neck of femur

(d) Posterior dislocation of the hip

Clinical presentation is suggestive of extracapsular fracture of femur.

Lateral border of foot is touching the couch means that there is free external rotation (as the fracture line is outside the capsule of hip joint) so that the lateral border of the foot is touching the couch.

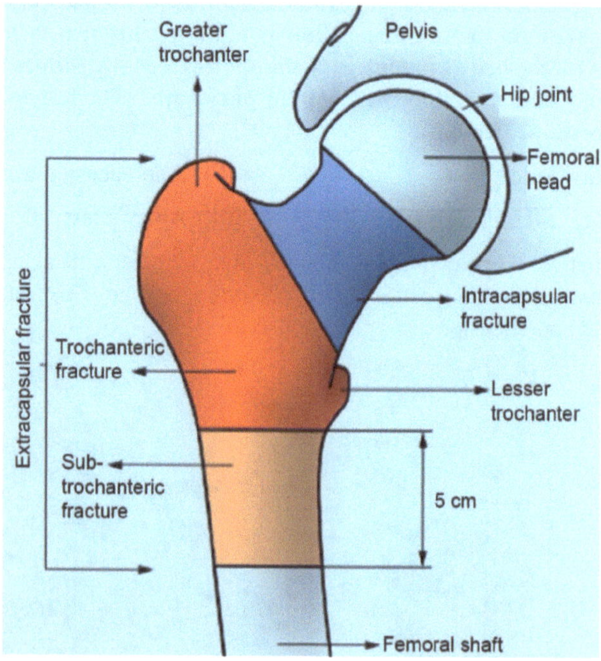

Answer: A i.e., Extracapsular fracture neck of femur

18. **An 80 years old female after fall was unable to walk. There was external rotation deformity. On examination SLR (straight leg raising) was not possible. There is broadening of greater trochanter and the lateral border of the foot is touching the couch. Most likely diagnosis:**

(a) Intracapsular fracture neck of femur

(b) Fracture intertrochanter

(c) Fracture subtrochanter

(d) Fracture greater trochanter

Clinical presentation is suggestive of fracture inter-trochanter.

SLR is not possible because of fracture.

Lateral border of foot is touching the couch means that there is free external rotation (as the fracture line is outside the capsule of hip joint)

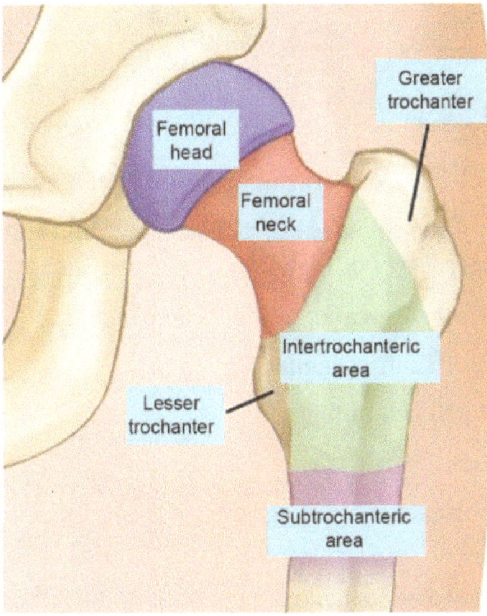

Answer: B i.e., Fracture intertrochanter

19. A 30 years old male was brought to the casualty following a road traffic accident. His physical examination revealed that his right lower limb was short, internally rotated, flexed and adducted at the hip. Most likely diagnosis:

(a) Fracture neck of femur

(b) Trochanteric fracture

(c) Central fracture dislocation of the hip

(d) Posterior dislocation of the hip

Clinical presentation is suggestive of posterior dislocation of the hip joint

FADIR (**F**lexion, **AD**duction, **I**nternal **R**otation) deformity is characteristic

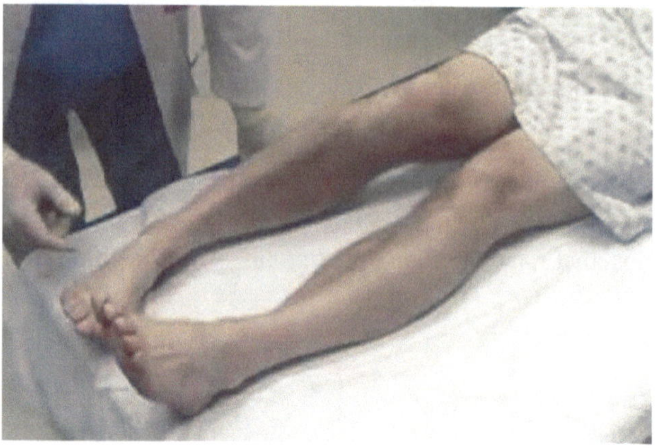

Answer: D i.e., Posterior dislocation of the hip

20. A patient with hip in adduction and medial rotation, is unable to move. Most likely diagnosis:

(a) Posterior dislocation of the head of femur

(b) Fracture shaft of femur

(c) Fracture neck of femur

(d) Sciatica

Clinical presentation is suggestive of posterior dislocation of the hip joint.

On X-ray, lesser trochanter is not seen on the affected side.

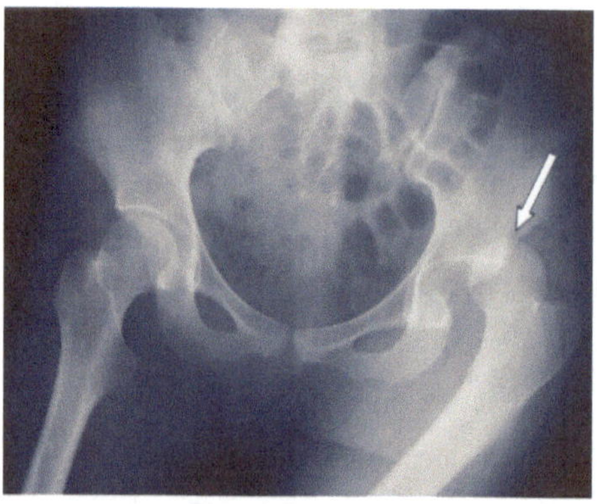

Answer: A i.e., Posterior dislocation of the head of femur

21. **Patient presented with flexion, adduction and internal rotation of lower limb after a road traffic accident suggest the diagnosis of:**

(a) Intracapsular fracture of the femoral neck

(b) Extracapsular fracture of the femoral neck

(c) Posterior dislocation of the hip

(d) Anterior dislocation of the hip

Clinical presentation is suggestive of posterior dislocation of the hip joint

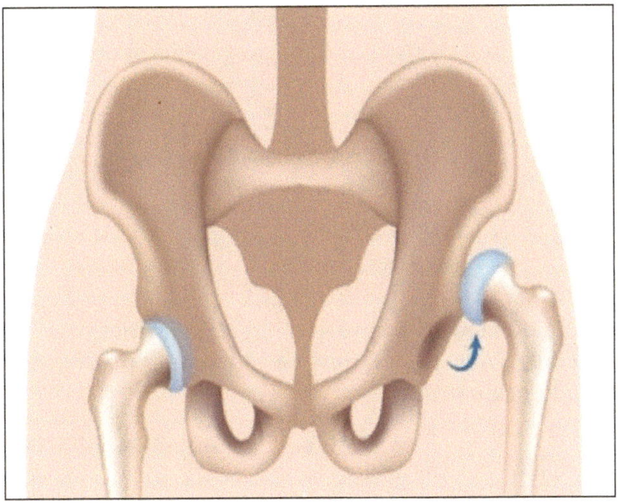

Answer: C i.e., Posterior dislocation of the hip

22. **A women aged 60 years suffers a fall. Her lower limb is extended and mildly externally rotated. Likely diagnosis:**

(a) Fracture neck of femur

(b) Intertrochanteric fracture

(c) Anterior dislocation of the hip

(d) Posterior dislocation of the hip

Clinical presentation is suggestive of fracture neck of femur.

Lower limb is mildly externally rotated as the fracture line is within the capsule of hip joint (intracapsular fracture), which prevents free external rotation of lower limb, as we see in intertrochanteric fractures (also known as extracapsular fracture).

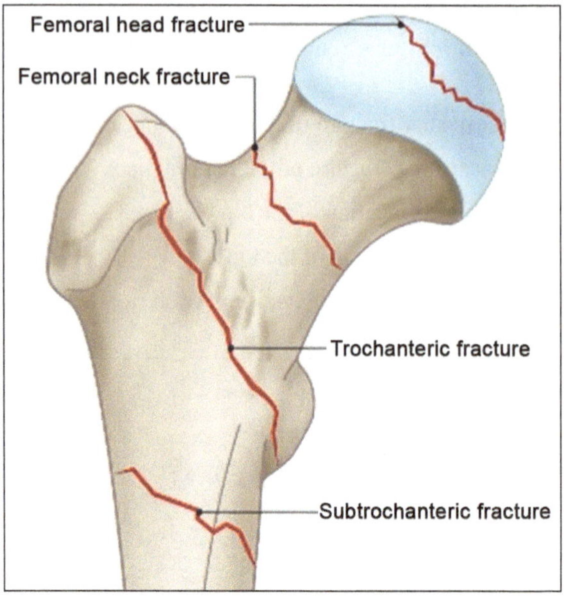

Answer: A i.e., Fracture neck of femur

23. **If a patient with a suspected fracture of the pelvis has some bleeding from the urethra and is unable to pass urine, what should be done next:**

(a) He should be encouraged to pass urine after being given antibiotics and analgesics

(b) He should be immediately catheterized in the ward

(c) A hot water bottle should be followed by injection of carbachol

(d) He should be prepared for surgery and catheterization attempted in the operation theatre

Clinical presentation is suggestive of rupture of urethra (as there is fracture of pelvis).

Catheterization is although contraindicated as this might further aggravate the rupture. Suprapubic cystostomy is preferred if a gentle attempt of catheterization fails.

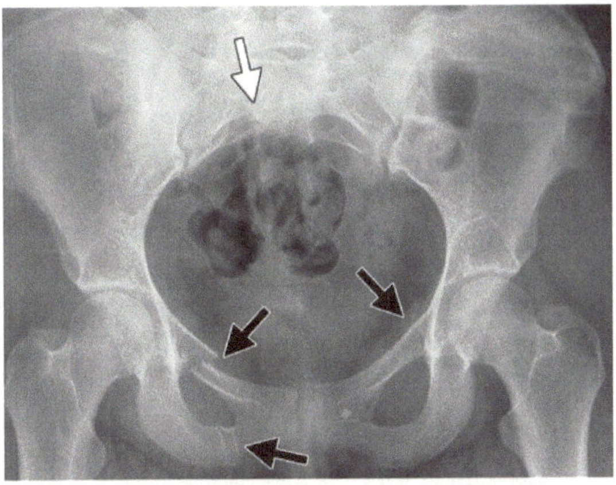

Answer: D i.e., He should be prepared for surgery and catheterization attempted in the operation theatre

24. Femoral neck fracture of three weeks old in a young patient is best managed by:

(a) Total hip replacement

(b) Reduction of fracture and femoral osteotomy

(c) Prosthetic replacement of femoral head

(d) Reduction of fracture and fixation with multiple pin or screw

In young patients, chances of fracture union are more (as compared to elderly) so internal fixation is preferred.

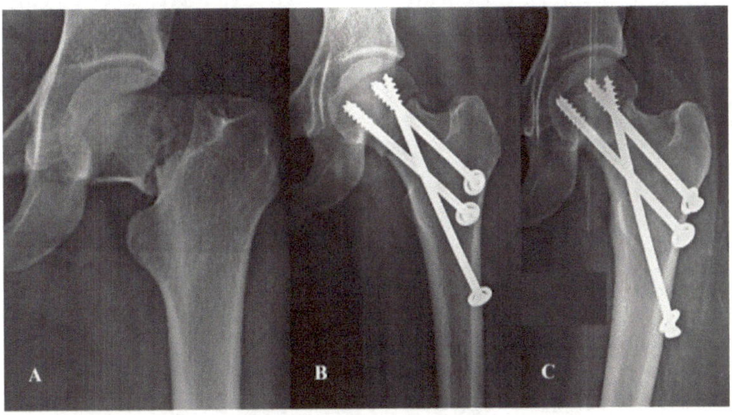

Answer: D i.e., Reduction of fracture and fixation with multiple pin or screw

25. Treatment of choice in fracture neck of femur in a 40 years old male presenting after 2 days:

(a) Hemiarthroplasty

(b) Closed reduction and internal fixation by cancellous screws

(c) Closed reduction and internal fixation by Austin Moore pins

(d) Plaster of Paris cats

In young patients, chances of fracture union are more (as compared to elderly) so internal fixation is preferred.

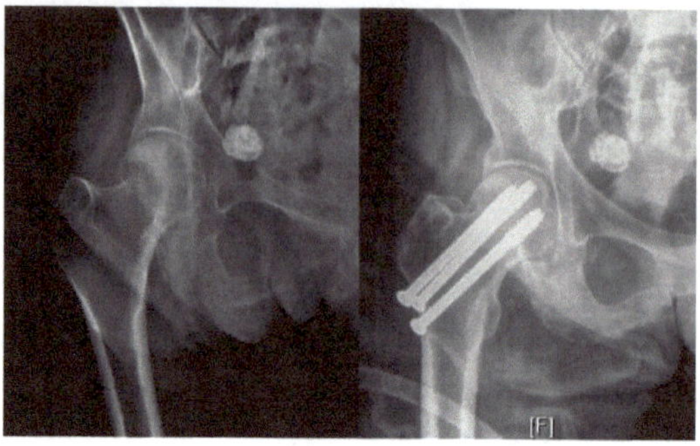

Answer: B i.e., Closed reduction and internal fixation by cancellous screws

26. In a 65 years old male with history of 6 weeks old, fracture neck of femur, is best managed by:

(a) Smith Peterson nailing

(b) McMurray's osteotomy

(c) Hemiarthroplasty

(d) Total hip replacement

In older patients, chances of fracture union are less (as compared to young) so hemi-replacement arthroplasty is preferred.

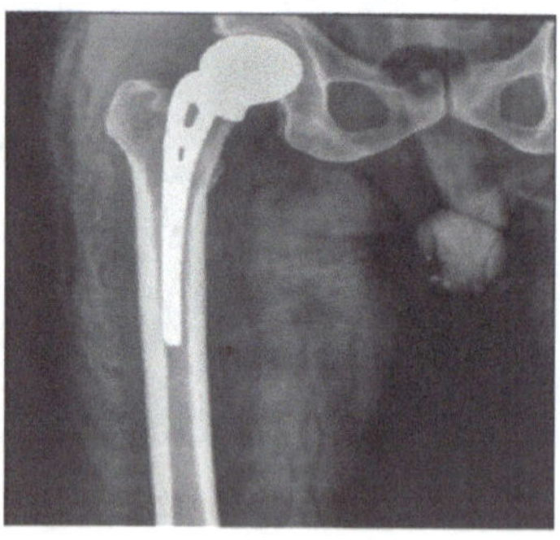

Answer: C i.e., Hemiarthroplasty

27. **An elderly woman was admitted with a fracture of the neck of right femur which failed to unite. On examination, an avascular necrosis/ AVN of the head of femur was noted. The condition would have resulted most probably from damage to:**

(a) Superior gluteal artery

(b) Inferior gluteal artery

(c) Acetabular branch of obturator artery

(d) Retinacular branches of circumflex femoral arteries

Clinical presentation is suggestive of injury to arterial blood supply to head of femur, which are torn during fracture neck of femur. That's why AVN of head of femur may develop despite operative fixation, as operation can fix the bone fragments but there is no surety that arterial supply would be regained.

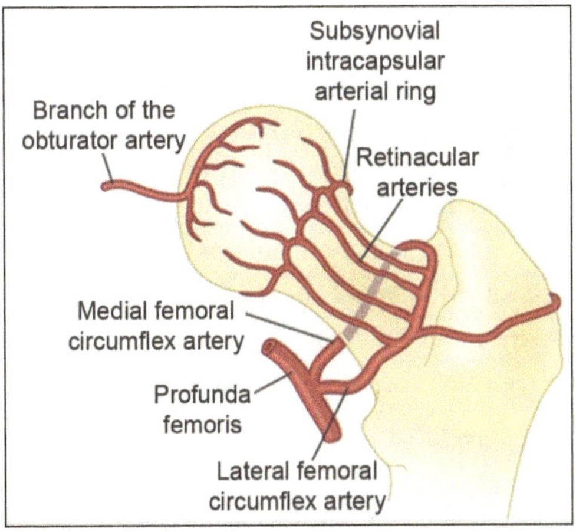

Answer: D i.e., Retinacular branches of circumflex femoral arteries

28. **An 18 years old boy was playing football, when he suddenly twisted his knee on the ankle and he fell down. He got up after 10 minutes and again started playing but next day, his knee was swollen and he could not move it. Most likely diagnosis:**

(a) Medial meniscus tear

(b) Anterior cruciate ligament tear

(c) Medial collateral ligament injury

(d) Posterior cruciate ligament injury

Clinical presentation is suggestive of medial meniscus tear

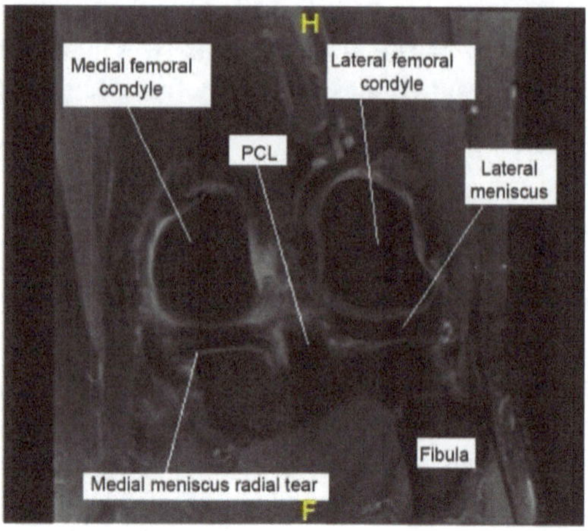

Answer: A i.e., Medial meniscus tear

29. **A 24 years old college student while playing hockey injured his right knee. This patient presented after 3 months with instability of knee joint in full extension without instability at 90 degrees of flexion. Structure most commonly damaged is:**
    (a) Anteromedial bundle of anterior cruciate ligament
    (b) Posteromedial bundle of anterior cruciate ligament
    (c) Posterior cruciate ligament
    (d) Anterior horn of lateral meniscus

Clinical presentation is suggestive of damage to posteromedial bundle of anterior cruciate ligament

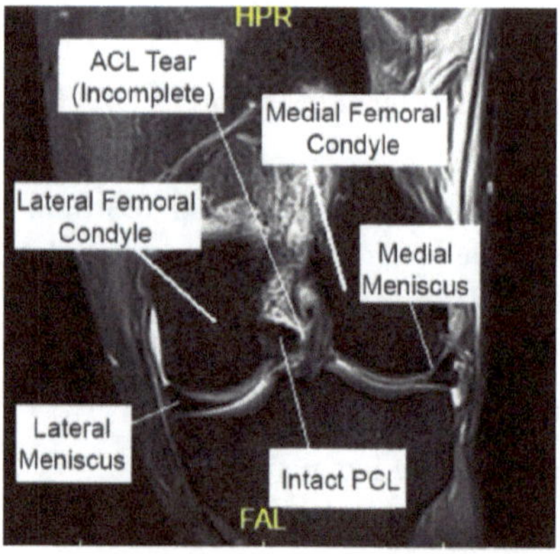

Answer: B i.e., Posteromedial bundle of anterior cruciate ligament

30. **Treatment of choice for non-united fracture of lower one-fourth tibia with multiple discharging sinuses and various puckered scar with 4 cm shortening of leg:**

(a) Plating (b) External fixator

(c) Ilizarov's fixator (d) Intramedullary nail

Clinical presentation is suggestive of non-union of fracture with chronic osteomyelitis and shortening.

Such a case is best managed with Ilizarov's fixator, which allows lengthening as well.

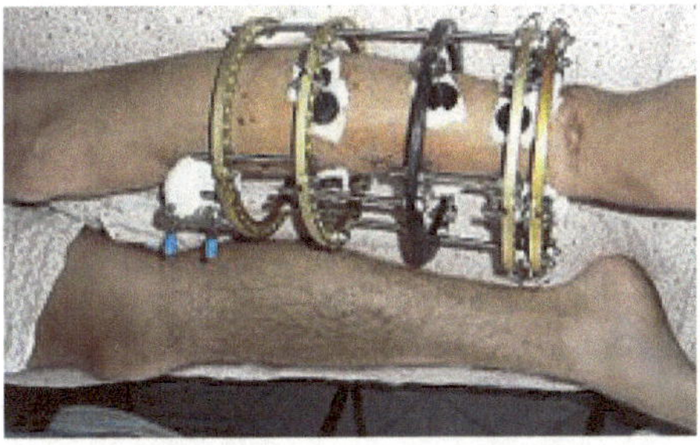

Answer: C i.e., Ilizarov's fixator

31. **A person comes with fracture of tibia with swelling of lower leg. Pulse is feeble but palpable. Intra-compartmental pressure was raised. Next step in management:**

(a) Fasciotomy (b) External fixation

(c) Lower limb venography (d) Interlock nailing

Clinical presentation is suggestive of impending compartment syndrome.

It is best managed by fasciotomy.

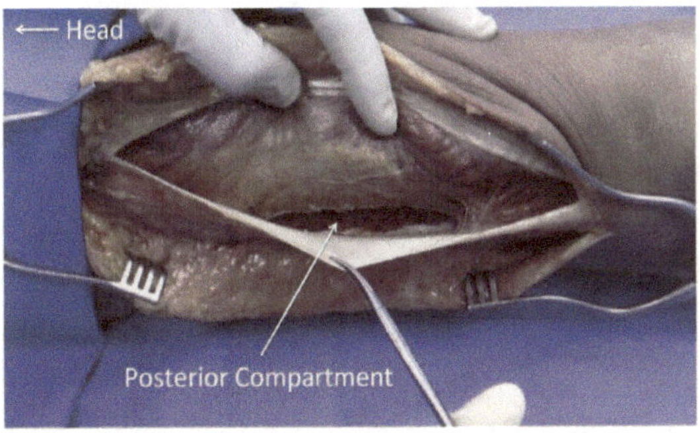

Answer: A i.e., Fasciotomy

32. A 46-years old, known alcoholic presented with pain in the dorsal spine. On examination, there is tenderness at the dorso-lumbar junction. Radiograph shows destruction of the 11th dorsal vertebra with loss of disc space between D11-D12 vertebra. Most likely diagnosis:

(a) Metastatic spine disease (b) Pott's spine

(c) Missed trauma (d) Multiple myeloma

Clinical presentation is suggestive of Pott's spine/ Tuberculosis of spine.

Loss of intervertebral disc space is an early sign of TB spine.

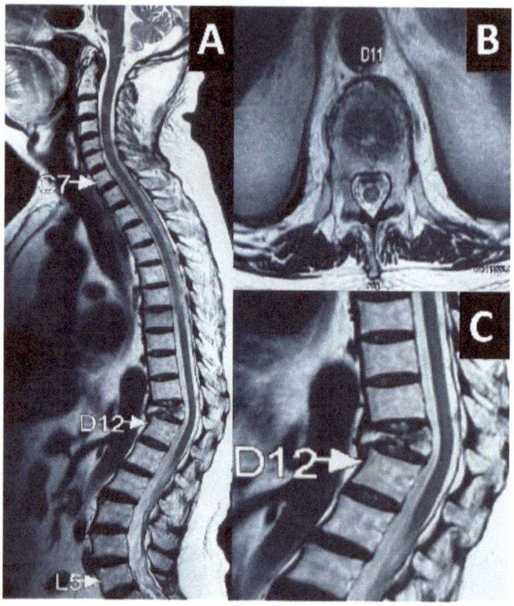

Answer: B i.e., Pott's spine

33. A patient presented with chronic discharging sinus through which bone particle comes out occasionally. Most likely diagnosis:

(a) Acute osteomyelitis (b) Subacute osteomyelitis

(c) Chronic osteomyelitis (d) Garre's osteomyelitis

Clinical presentation is suggestive of chronic OM.

Discharge of bony spicules through the sinuses is diagnostic of chronic OM.

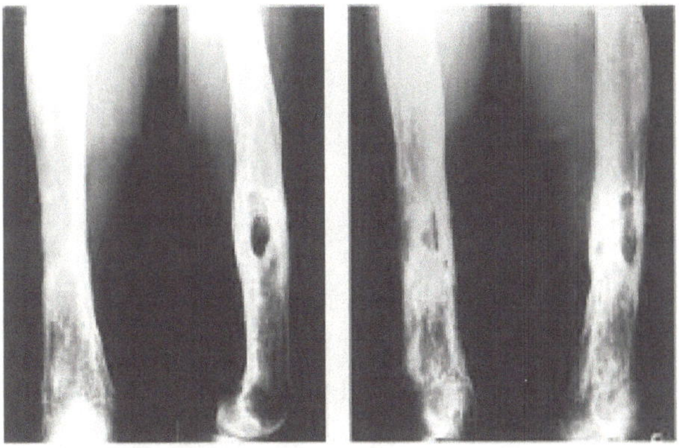

Answer: C i.e., Chronic osteomyelitis

34. **An 8 years old boy presents with gradually progressing swelling and pain since, 6 months over the upper tibia. On X-ray, there is a lytic lesion with sclerotic margins in the upper tibial metaphysis. Most likely diagnosis:**

(a) Osteogenic sarcoma (b) Osteoclastoma

(c) Brodie's abscess (d) Ewing's sarcoma

Clinical presentation is suggestive of Brodie's abscess

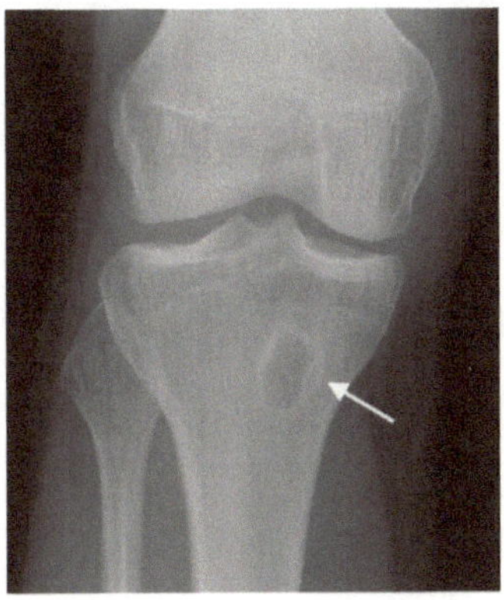

Answer: C i.e., Brodie's abscess

35. **A 35 years old lady had chronic backache. On X-ray, she had a D12 vertebra collapse, but intervertebral disc space is maintained. All are possible EXCEPT:**

(a) Multiple myeloma (b) Osteoporosis

(c) Metastasis (d) Tuberculosis

In TB spine, there is reduction in intervertebral disc space.

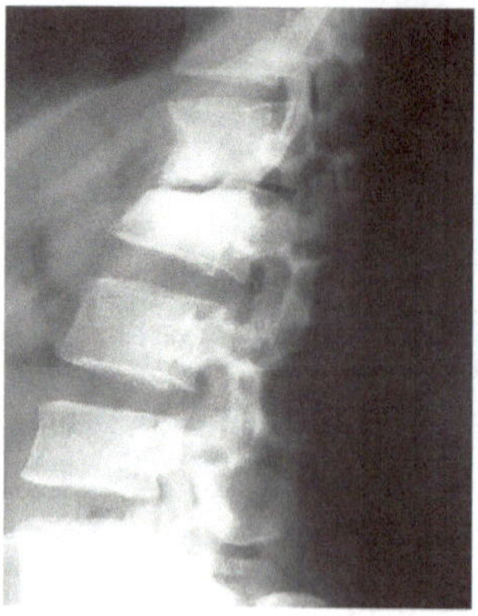

Answer: D i.e., Tuberculosis

36. A 7-years old comes with fever and tibial swelling. X-ray shows periosteal reaction. Laboratory result shows raised ESR and leucocytosis. What is the next step in diagnosis of the patient:

(a) MRI (b) Pus culture

(c) Bone biopsy (d) Blood culture

Clinical presentation is suggestive of acute osteomyelitis.

Blood culture can yield the causative organism in many cases, against which we can start the appropriate antibiotic (as per sensitivity report)

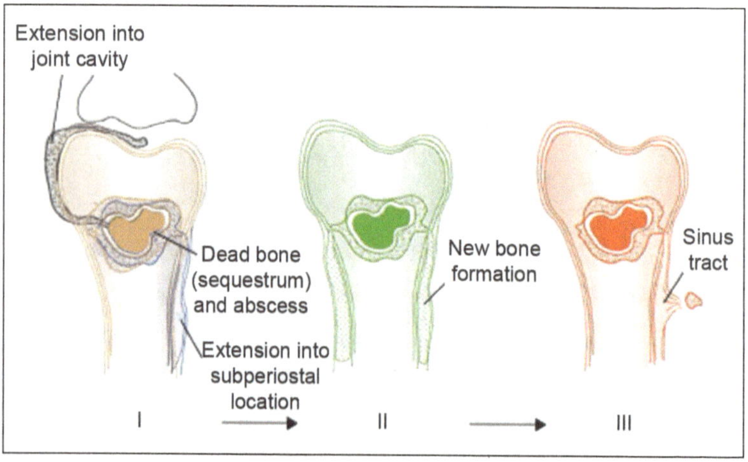

Answer: D i.e., Blood culture

37. Babu, a 19 years old male has a small circumscribed sclerotic swelling over diaphysis of femur. Most likely diagnosis:

(a) Osteoclastoma (b) Osteosarcoma

(c) Ewing sarcoma (d) Osteoid osteoma

Clinical presentation is suggestive of osteoid osteoma.

An osteoid osteoma is a noncancerous (benign) bone tumor. Each tumor usually measures less than 1 inch across. These tumors don't grow or spread anywhere else.

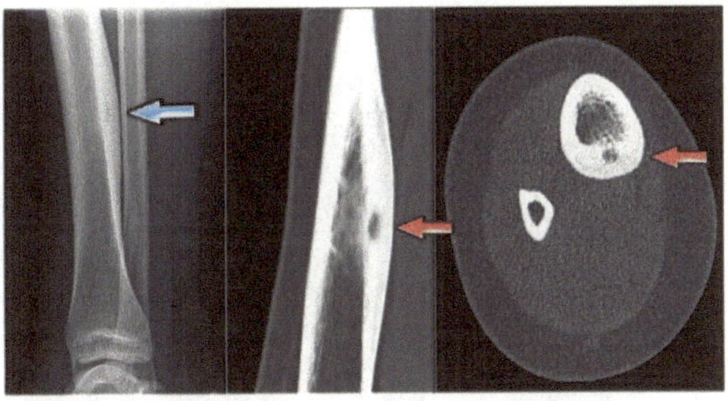

Answer: D i.e., Osteoid osteoma

38. A 7 years old child presents with a lesion in the upper tibia. X-ray shows radiolucent area with Codman's triangle and Sunray appearance. Most likely diagnosis:

(a) Ewing sarcoma (b) Osteosarcoma

(c) Osteoid osteoma (d) Chondrosarcoma

Clinical presentation is suggestive of osteosarcoma.

Osteosarcoma is a rare type of bone cancer in which malignant (cancerous) cells produce irregular bone.

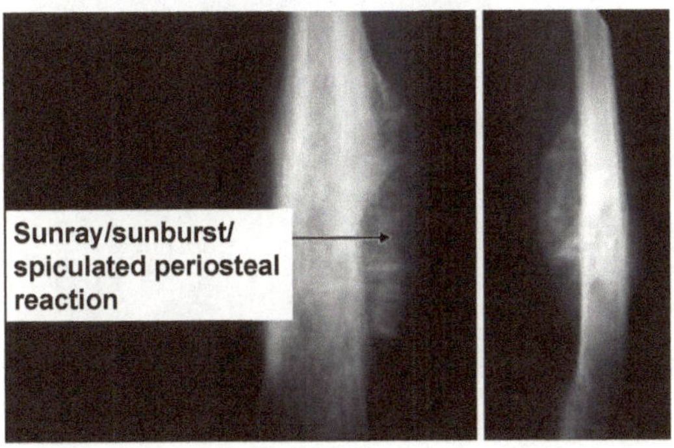

Answer: B i.e., Osteosarcoma

39. A patient presents with pain in the thigh, relieved by aspirin. X-ray shows a radiolucent mass surrounded by sclerosis. Most likely diagnosis:

(a) Osteoma (b) Osteoid osteoma

(c) Osteoblastoma (d) Osteoclastoma

Clinical presentation is suggestive of osteoid osteoma.

Pain of osteoid osteoma is relieved by Aspirin therefore it is also known as aspirin tumor.

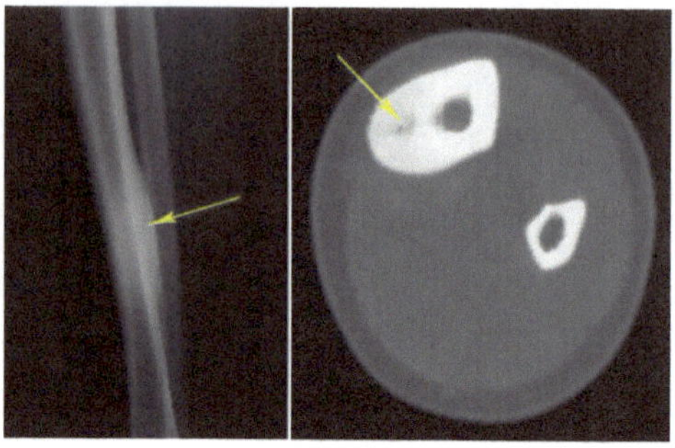

Answer: B i.e., Osteoid osteoma

40. A 10 years old child presented with mid-tibial swelling which X-ray revealed a lytic lesion with sclerotic margins. Most likely diagnosis:

(a) Osteoid osteoma (b) Eosinophilic granuloma

(c) Fibrous cortical defect (d) Fibrous dysplasia

Clinical presentation is suggestive of osteoid osteoma.

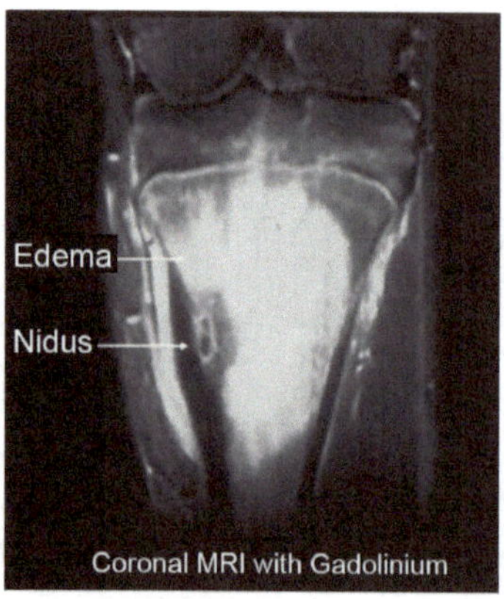

Coronal MRI with Gadolinium

Answer: A i.e., Osteoid osteoma

41. **A 12 years old girl complains of pain persisting in her right thigh for several weeks with low grade fever. Radiograph reveals a mass in the diaphyseal region of the left femur with overlying cortical erosion and soft tissue extension. A biopsy of the lesion shows numerous small round cells, rich is PAS positive diastase sensitive granules. Most likely diagnosis:**

(a) Osteogenic sarcoma

(b) Osteoblastoma

(c) Ewing's sarcoma

(d) Chondrosarcoma

Clinical presentation is suggestive of Ewing's sarcoma.

Ewing sarcoma (ES) is an aggressive tumor of adolescents and young adults, which constitutes 10% to 15% of all bone sarcomas.

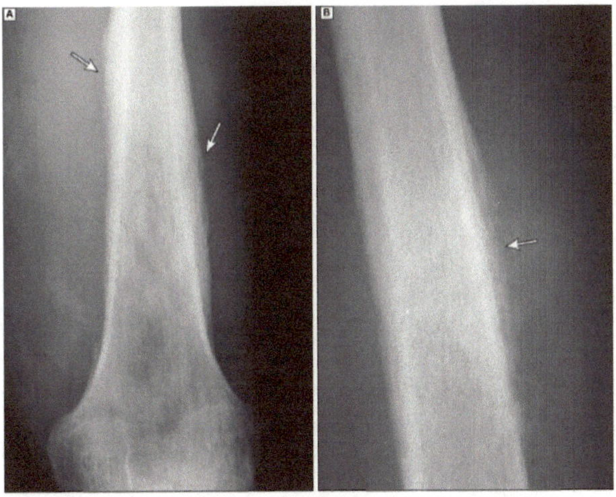

Answer: C i.e., Ewing's sarcoma

42. **A 15-years old boy is injured while playing cricket. X-rays of the leg rule out possibility of a fracture. However, the radiologist reports that the boy has an evidence of an aggressive bony tumour with bone destruction and soft tissue mass. The bone biopsy reveals a bone cancer with neural differentiation. Most likely diagnosis:**

(a) Chondroblastoma (b) Ewing's sarcoma

(c) Neuroblastoma (d) Osteosarcoma

Clinical presentation is suggestive of Ewing's sarcoma.

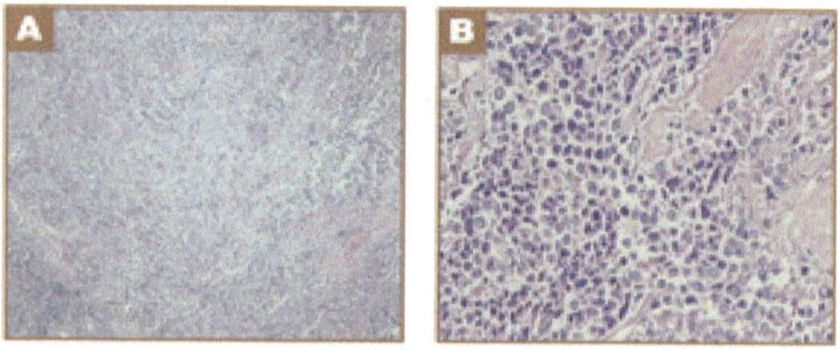

Answer: B i.e., Ewing's sarcoma

43. A young girl presented with swelling of right thigh, with history of trauma 2 months back. Now she presents with swelling at mid-shaft of femur and low-grade fever. ESR is mildly elevated. X-rays shows a laminated periosteal reaction. Next line of investigation:

(a) MRI

(b) Biopsy

(c) Bone scan

(d) Blood count & C-reactive protein

Clinical presentation is suggestive of Ewing's sarcoma

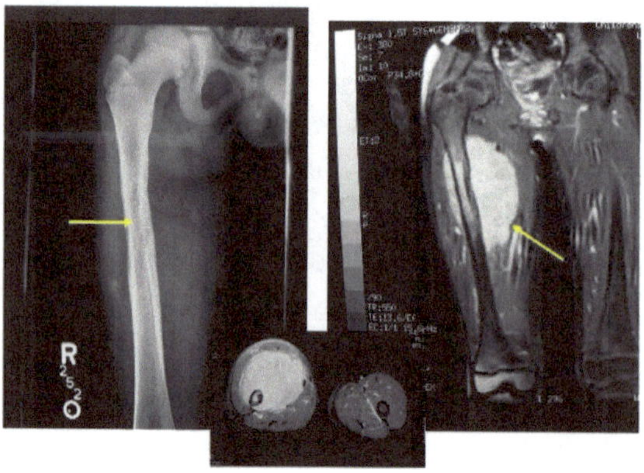

Answer: A i.e., MRI

44. A 15 years-old boy presented with painful swelling over the left shoulder. Radiograph of the shoulder showed an osteolytic area with stippled calcification over the proximal humeral epiphysis. Biopsy of the lesion revealed an immature, fibrous matrix with scattered giant cells. Most likely diagnosis:

(a) Giant cell tumour (b) Chondroblastoma

(c) Osteosarcoma (d) Chondromyxoid fibroma

Clinical presentation is suggestive of chondroblastoma.

Chondroblastoma, also called a calcifying giant cell tumor or Codman tumor is a rare, non-cancerous tumor made up of a mass of cartilage tissue.

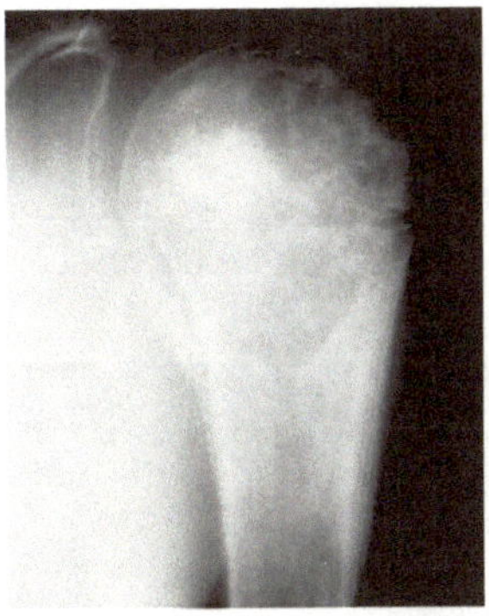

Answer: B i.e., Chondroblastoma

45. A 45 years male presented with an expansile lesion in the centre of femoral metaphysis. The lesion shows endosteal scalloping and punctuate calcifications. Most likely diagnosis:

(a) Osteosarcoma (b) Chondrosarcoma

(c) Simple bone cyst (d) Fibrous dysplasia

Clinical presentation is suggestive of chondrosarcoma.

Chondrosarcomas are a heterogeneous group of malignant bone tumors that share in common the production of chondroid (cartilaginous) matrix

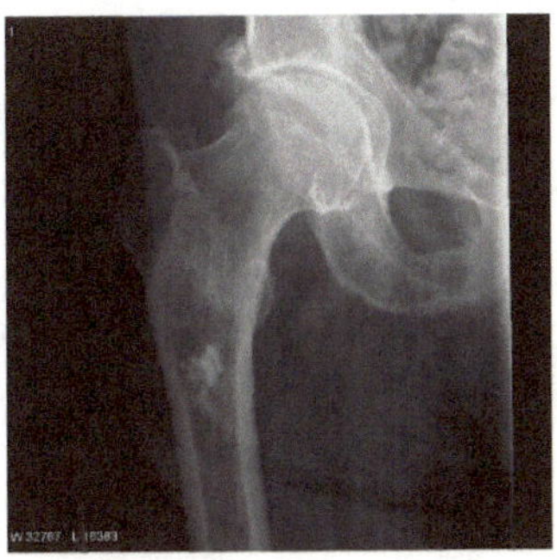

Answer: B i.e., Chondrosarcoma

46. A 33-years old man presented with a slowly progressive swelling in the middle one-third of his right tibia. X-ray examination revealed multiple sharply demarcated radiolucent lesions separated by areas of dense and sclerotic bone. Microscopic examination of a biopsy specimen revealed island of epithelial cells in a fibrous stroma. Most likely diagnosis:

(a) Adamantinoma (b) Osteofibrous dysplasia

(c) Osteosarcoma (d) Fibrous cortical defect

Clinical presentation is suggestive of adamantinoma.

Adamantinoma is a rare low-grade malignant bone tumor of uncertain histogenesis, which occurs commonly in the diaphyses and metaphyses of the tibia.

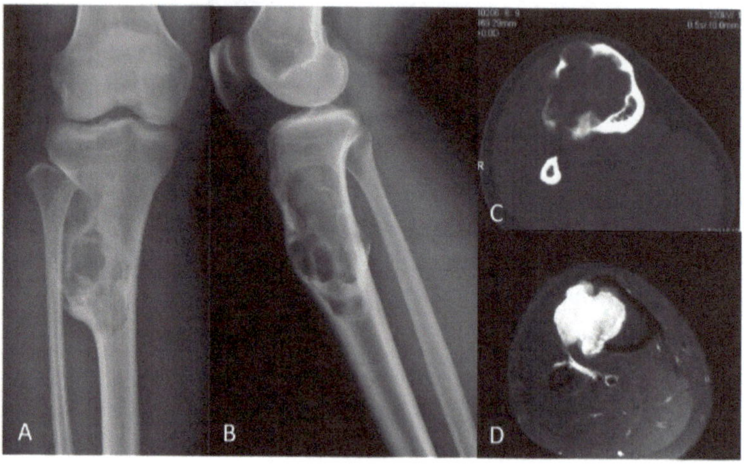

Answer: A i.e., Adamantinoma

47. Skull X-ray of a patient shows lytic bevelled lesion. Most likely diagnosis:

(a) Multiple myeloma (b) Eosinophilic granuloma

(c) Metastasis (d) Osteosarcoma

Clinical presentation is suggestive of eosinophilic granuloma.

Eosinophilic granuloma of the bone is a rare, noncancerous tumor that tends to affect children.

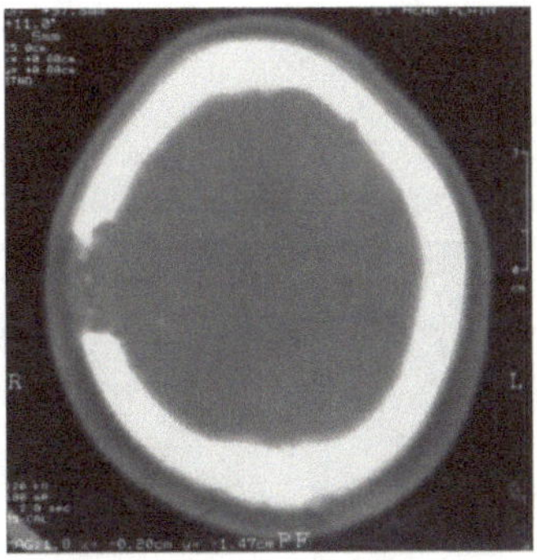

Answer: B i.e., Eosinophilic granuloma

48. **A 50-years old patient presents with long standing backache. Skiagram shows lesion in the midline involving the sacrum, which is lytic and expansile. Most likely diagnosis:**

(a) Chordoma (b) Synovial sarcoma

(c) Osteoclastoma (d) Fibrosarcoma

Clinical presentation is suggestive of chordoma.

Chordoma is a rare slow-growing neoplasm thought to arise from cellular remnants of the notochord.

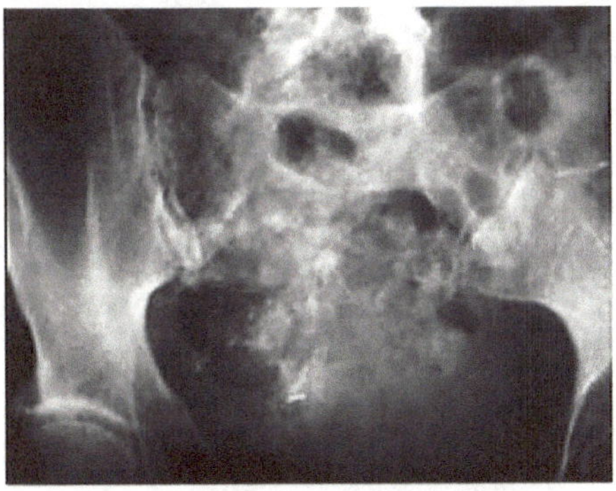

Answer: A i.e., Chordoma

49. **Ramu, an 11-years old boy presented with pain in the arm. On X-ray, his upper end of humerus demonstrates an expansile lesion in the metaphysis with breach of the overlying cortex. Most likely diagnosis:**

(a) Aneurysmal bone cyst (b) Unicameral bone cyst

(c) Chondroblastoma (d) Osteoclastoma

Clinical presentation is suggestive of aneurysmal bone cyst.

An aneurysmal bone cyst is a benign, blood-filled lesion in the bone that tends to expand or grow. While it is referred to as a cyst, it is a true benign bone tumor surrounded by a thin wall of bone.

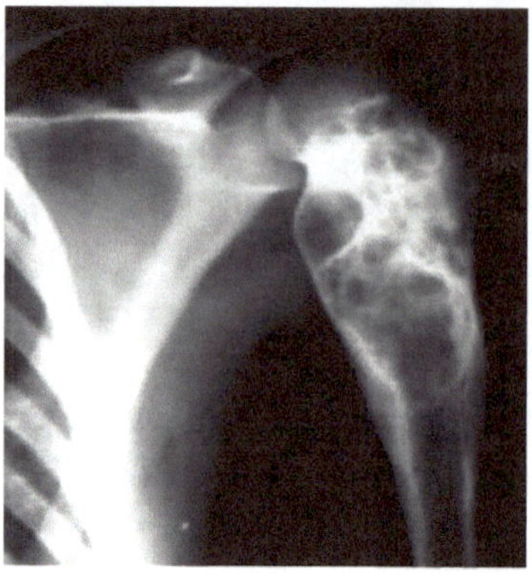

Answer: A i.e., Aneurysmal bone cyst

50. Babloo, a 10-years old boy presented with fracture of humerus. X-ray revealed a lytic lesion at the upper end. Most likely diagnosis:

(a) Unicameral bone cyst
(b) Osteosarcoma
(c) Osteoclastoma
(d) Aneurysmal bone cyst

Clinical presentation is suggestive of unicameral bone cyst.

Unicameral bone cysts are fluid-filled spaces inside bone. The word unicameral means "one chamber" and describes the single fluid-filled chamber in each cyst. It can lead to pathological fracture.

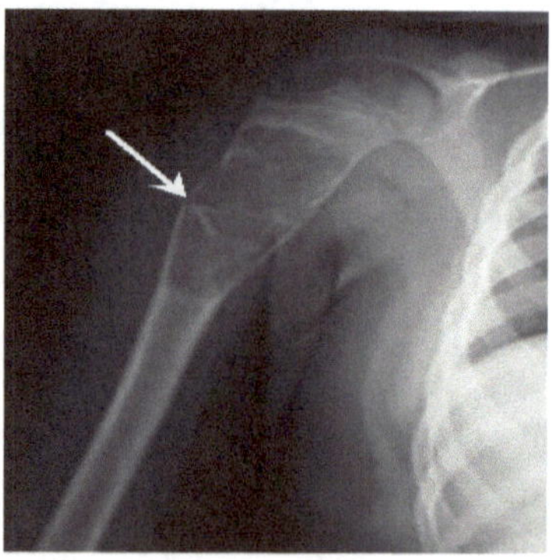

Answer: A i.e., Unicameral bone cyst

51. A 60 years old male has back pain and vertebral collapse. Most likely diagnosis:

(a) TB spine

(b) Ankylosing spondylitis

(c) Secondaries in spine

(d) Intervertebral disc prolapse

Clinical presentation is suggestive of secondaries/ metastasis to spine.

Spinal metastases form when cancer spreads to the spine from another area in the body (metastasizes)

C

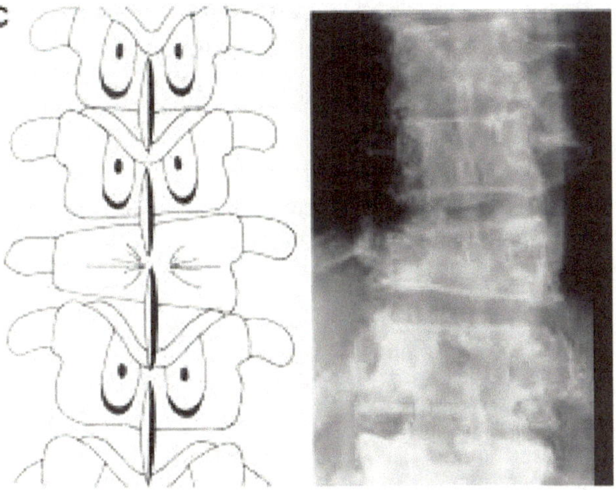

Answer: C i.e., Secondaries in spine

52. A patient developed paraplegia. On routine examination and X-ray, it was found that there was osteoblastic lesion in the spine. Most likely cause of such a presentation:

(a) Carcinoma thyroid

(b) Carcinoma prostate

(c) Carcinoma breast

(d) Carcinoma pancreas

Clinical presentation is suggestive of carcinoma prostate.

Osteoblastic metastases develop when cancer cells invade the bone and cause too many bone cells to form. The bone becomes very dense (sclerotic). Osteoblastic metastases often happen when prostate cancer spreads to the bone.

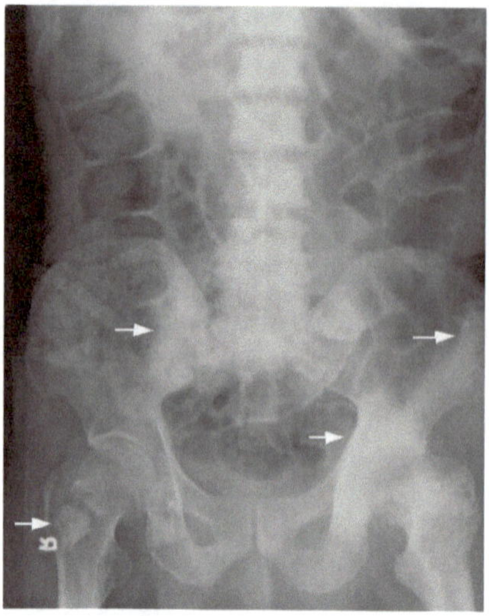

Answer: B i.e., Carcinoma prostate

53. A male patient had expansile, lytic, osseous metastasis in bone. Most likely primary malignancy is in:

(a) Kidney (b) Bronchus

(c) Breast (d) Prostate

Clinical presentation is suggestive of bony metastasis from renal cancers.

Osteolytic metastases develop when metastatic cancer cells break down too much of the bone, making it very weak.

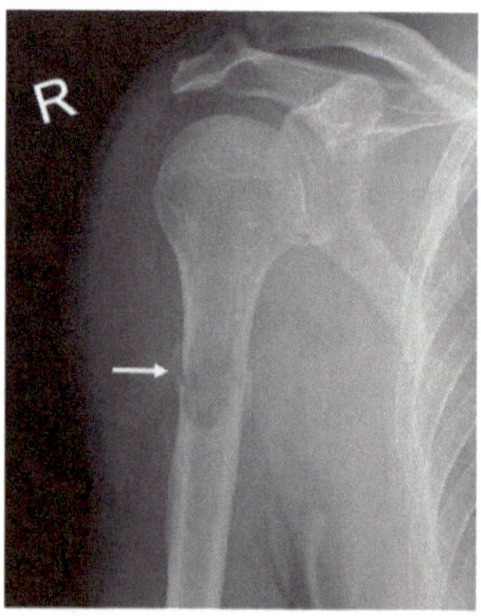

Answer: A i.e., Kidney

54. A 60 years old male with bony abnormality at upper tibia associated with sensorineural deafness. On laboratory examination, serum alkaline phosphatase levels are 440 IU/ ml, elevated serum calcium and normal phosphate levels. Skeletal survey shows ivory vertebrae and cotton wool spots on X-ray skull. Most likely diagnosis:

(a) Fibrous dysplasia (b) Paget's disease

(c) Osteosclerotic metastasis (d) Osteoporosis

Clinical presentation is suggestive of Paget's disease.

Paget's disease of bone disrupts the normal cycle of bone renewal, causing bones to become weakened and possibly deformed.

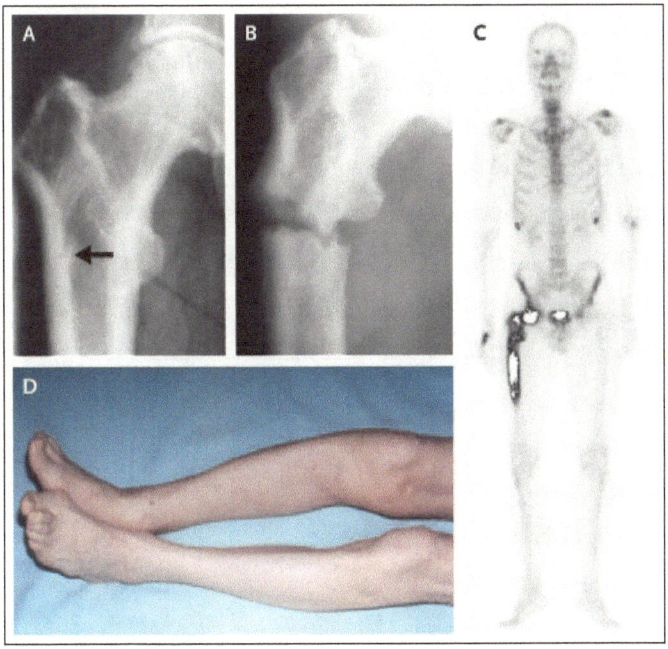

Answer: B i.e., Paget's disease

55. A patient of leprosy presented with clumsiness of hand. Clumsiness is due to palsy of which muscle:

(a) Extensor carpi ulnaris (b) Abductor pollicis brevis

(c) Opponens pollicis (d) Interossei muscles

Clinical presentation is suggestive of paralysis of interossei muscles.

All the interossei muscles are supplied by ulnar nerve.

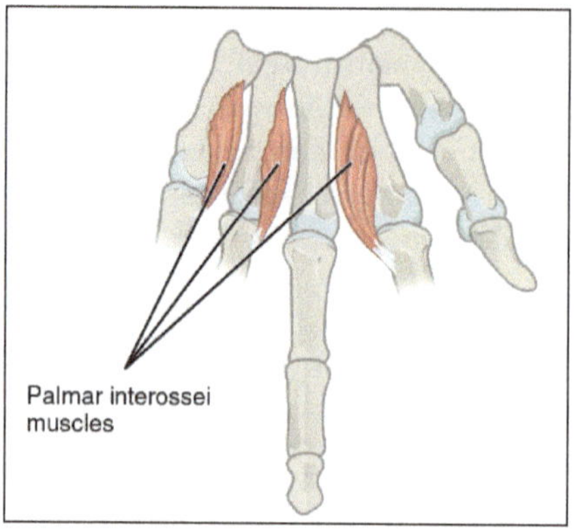

Answer: D i.e., Interosseous muscle

56. **Following an incised wound in front of the wrist, the subject is unable to oppose the tips of the little finger and the thumb. Nerve involved are:**

(a) Ulnar nerve (b) Median nerve

(c) Musculocutaneous nerve (d) Radial nerve

Clinical presentation is suggestive of paralysis of median nerve.

Muscle paralyzed is opponens pollicis and the movement lost is opposition.

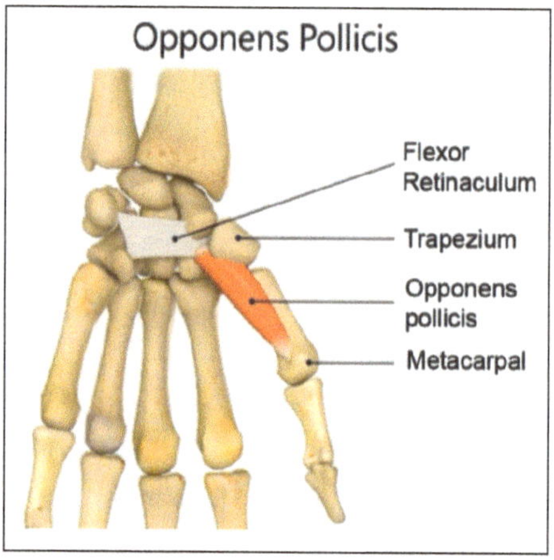

Answer: B i.e., Median nerve

57. **A boy presents with complains of hypoaesthesia and wasting of thenar eminence. The nerve most likely to be damaged in this patient:**

(a) Musculocutaneous nerve (b) Median nerve
(c) Ulnar nerve (d) Radial nerve

Clinical presentation is suggestive of median nerve palsy.

The majority of the thenar muscles are innervated by the median nerve (T1). The exceptions are the deep head of flexor pollicis brevis and adductor pollicis muscle that receive their innervation via the ulnar nerve (C8, T1).

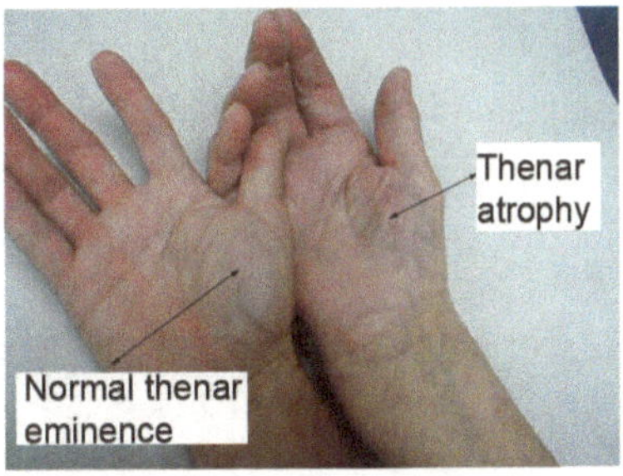

Answer: B i.e., Median nerve

58. A 56-years old female presents with nocturnal pain in the right thumb, index and middle fingers for the past 3 months. All the provocative tests can be performed EXCEPT:

(a) Finkelstein's test (b) Tinel sign
(c) Phalen's test (d) Tourniquet's test

Clinical presentation is suggestive of Carpal tunnel syndrome

Finkelstein's test is done for DeQuervain's tenosynovitis.

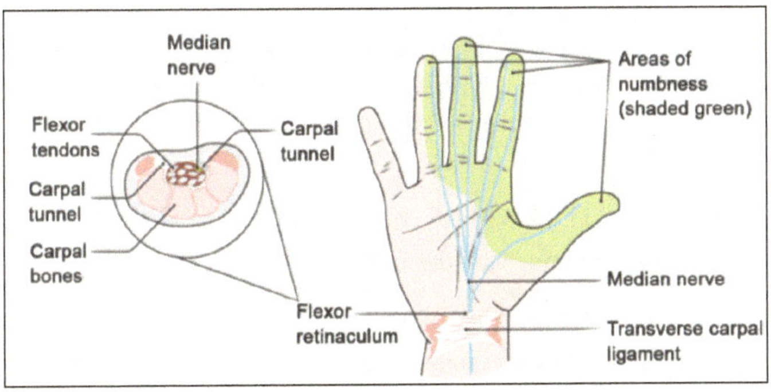

Answer: A i.e., Finkelstein's test

59. A young boy who was driving motorcycle at a high speed collided with a tree and was thrown on his right shoulder. Though there

was no fracture but later on his right arm was medially rotated and pronated. Following facts are correct regarding this patient EXCEPT:

(a) The injury was at Erb's point

(b) A lesion of C5 and C6 was present

(c) The median and ulnar nerves were affected

(d) Supraspinatus, infraspinatus, subclavius and biceps brachii were paralyzed

Clinical presentation is suggestive of Erb's palsy.

Erb's palsy is a paralysis of the arm caused by injury to the upper group of the arm›s main nerves, specifically the severing of the upper trunk C5–C6.

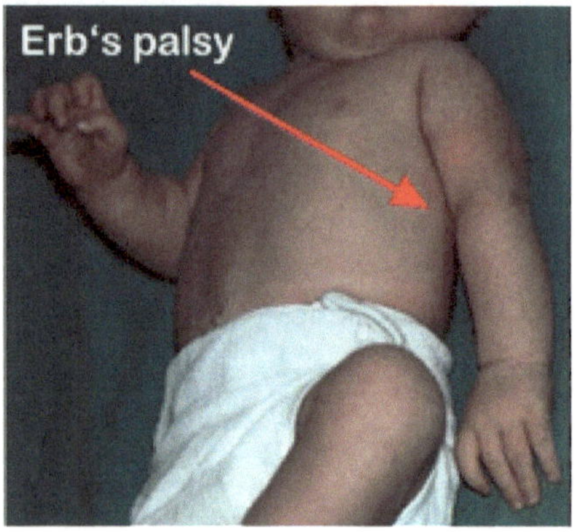

Answer: C i.e., The median and ulnar nerves were affected

60. **A 30-years old male underwent excision of the right radial head. Following surgery, the patient developed inability to extend the fingers and thumb of the right hand. He did not have any sensory deficit. Most likely diagnosis:**

(a) Injury to posterior interosseous nerve

(b) Iatrogenic injury to common extensor origin

(c) Injury to anterior interosseous nerve

(d) High radial nerve palsy

Clinical presentation is suggestive of finger drop, which is due to paralysis of posterior interosseous nerve (branch of radial nerve)

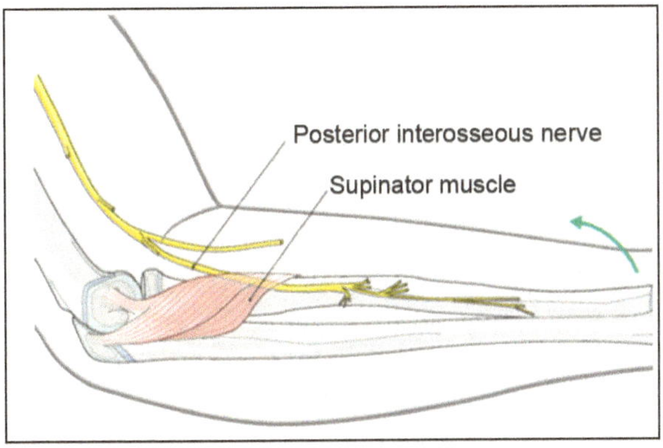

Answer: A i.e., Injury to posterior interosseous nerve

61. A young female presented with bony pain. She had raised serum alkaline phosphatase and raised parathormone level along with low calcium and low phosphate level. Most likely diagnosis:

(a) Primary hyperparathyroidism (b) Paget's disease

(c) Osteoporosis (d) Vitamin D deficiency

Clinical presentation is suggestive of osteomalacia.

Osteomalacia describes a disorder of "bone softening" in adults that is usually due to prolonged deficiency of vitamin D.

Disease	Calcium	Phosphate	25-OH Vitamin D	Parathyroid Hormone	Alkaline Phosphatase (Bone)
Osteoporosis	N	N	N	N	N
Osteomalacia or rickets owing to malabsorption or dietary lack	Low–N	Low–N	Decreased	Increased–N	Increased
Osteomalacia with renal bone disease	Variable	N–Increased	Variable	Increased–N	Increased
Familial hypo-phosphataemic rickets	N	Decreased	N	N	Increased
Primary hyperpara-thyroidism	Increased	Decreased–N	N	Increased–high N	Increased
Paget's disease	N	N	N	N	Increased

Answer: D i.e., Vitamin D deficiency

62. During a routine check-up, a 67 years old man is found to have a level of serum alkaline phosphatase three times the upper limit

of normal. Serum calcium and phosphate concentrations and liver function test results are normal. He is asymptomatic. Most likely diagnosis:

(a) Metastatic bone disease

(b) Primary hyperparathyroidism

(c) Paget's disease of the bone

(d) Osteomalacia

Clinical presentation is suggestive of osteomalacia.

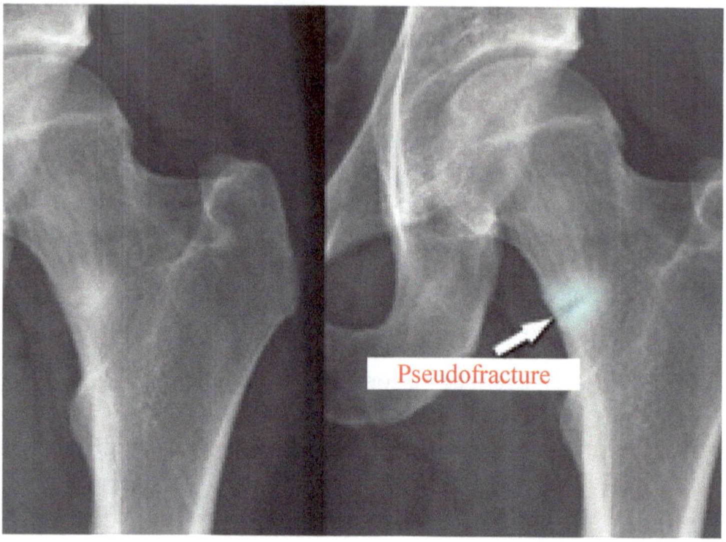

Answer: D i.e., Osteomalacia

63. **A 50 years old man presented with multiple pathological fractures. His serum calcium was 11.5 mg/ dl and phosphate were 2.5 gm/ dl. Alkaline phosphate was 940 IU/ dl. Most likely diagnosis:**

(a) Osteoporosis (b) Osteomalacia

(c) Multiple myeloma (d) Hyperparathyroidism

Clinical presentation is suggestive of hyperparathyroidism (excess of parathormone).

Normal serum calcium level is 9-11 mg/ dl.

Bone Disease	Ca^{++}	Phosphate	Alkaline Phosphatase
Osteoporosis	Normal	Normal	Normal
Osteomalacia	↓	↓	↑
Paget's	Normal	Normal	↑↑
Myeloma	↑	↑, Normal	Normal
Bone Metastasis	↑	↑, Normal	↑
1° Hyperparathyroidism	↑	↓, Normal	Normal, ↑
Hypoparathyroidism	↓	↑	Normal
Renal Failure	↓	↑	Normal, ↑

Answer: D i.e., Hyperparathyroidism

64. A young patient presents with enlargement of costo-chondral junction and with the white line of Frenkel at metaphysis. Most likely diagnosis:

(a) Scurvy
(b) Rickets
(c) Osteomalacia
(d) Hyperparathyroidism

Clinical presentation is suggestive of scurvy.

Scurvy happens when there is a lack of vitamin C, or ascorbic acid. The deficiency leads to symptoms of weakness, anemia, gum disease, and skin problems.

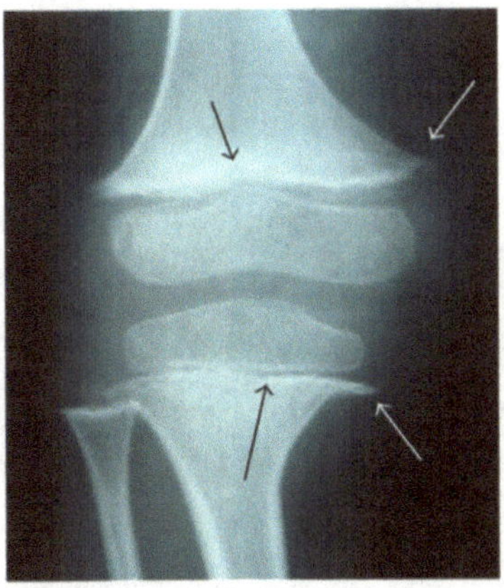

Answer: A i.e., Scurvy

65. A 40 years old man presented with acute onset of pain and swelling of left great toe. Urate crystals could be seen from the joint aspirate. Most likely diagnosis:

(a) Gout (b) Rheumatoid arthritis

(c) Psoriatic arthritis (d) Reiter's syndrome

Clinical presentation is suggestive of gout.

Gout is characterized by sudden, severe attacks of pain, swelling, redness and tenderness in one or more joints, most often in the big toe.

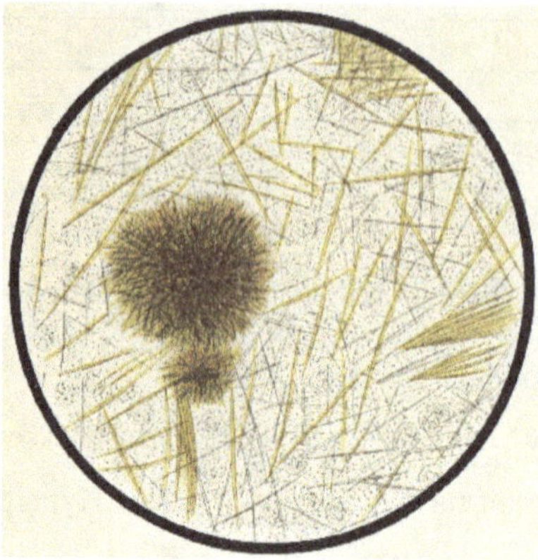

Answer: A i.e., Gout

66. **A 40 years old female present with multiple lytic bone lesions, fracture clavicle, periosteal resorption of 2nd and 3rd metacarpals. Most likely diagnosis:**

(a) Renal osteodystrophy (b) Osteomalacia

(c) Hyperparathyroidism (d) Hypoparathyroidism

Clinical presentation is suggestive of hyperparathyroidism

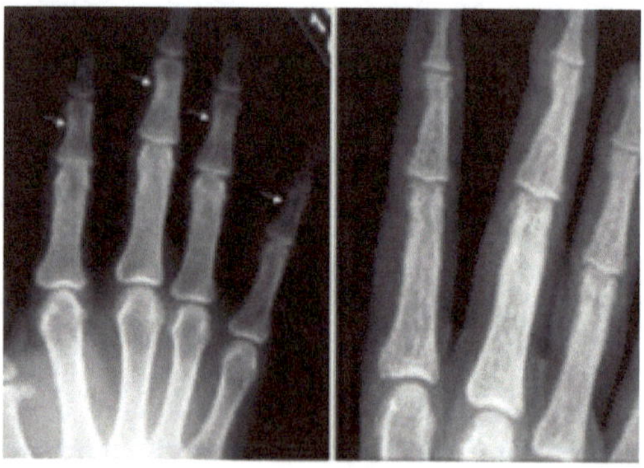

Answer: C i.e., Hyperparathyroidism

67. Young male having pain with morning stiffness of spine for 30 minutes and reduced chest movements. Most likely diagnosis:

(a) Ankylosing spondylitis

(b) Rheumatoid arthritis

(c) Gouty arthritis

(d) Osteoarthritis

Clinical presentation is suggestive of AS.

Ankylosing spondylitis is a form of painful, ongoing joint inflammation (chronic inflammatory arthritis) that primarily affects the spine.

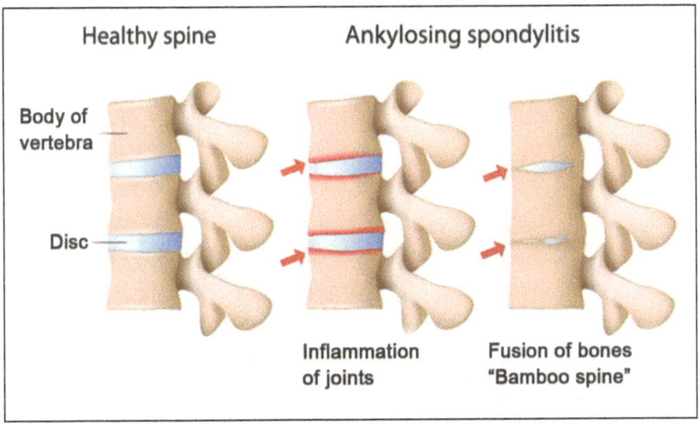

Answer: A i.e., Ankylosing spondylitis

68. A lady having flexion at proximal interphalangeal joint and hyperextension at distal interphalangeal joint of index finger is called:

(a) Boutonniere deformity

(b) Swan neck deformity

(c) Wind swept deformity

(d) Z-deformity

Clinical presentation is suggestive of Boutonniere deformity, which is seen in rheumatoid arthritis.

Boutonniere deformity is a deformity of the fingers in which the proximal interphalangeal joint (PIP) is flexed and the distal interphalangeal joint (DIP) is extended.

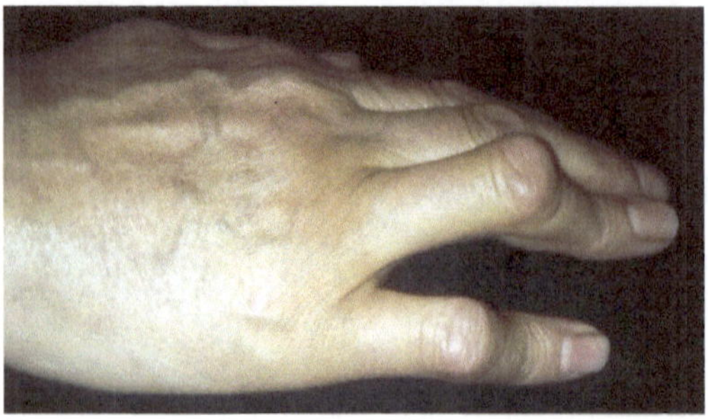

Answer: A i.e., Boutonniere deformity

69. **In a middle-aged male having back pain, syndesmophytes involving 4 continuous vertebrae are seen on X-ray. Most likely diagnosis:**

(a) Alkaptonuria
(b) Ankylosing spondylitis
(c) Rheumatoid arthritis
(d) Osteoarthritis

Clinical presentation is suggestive of AS

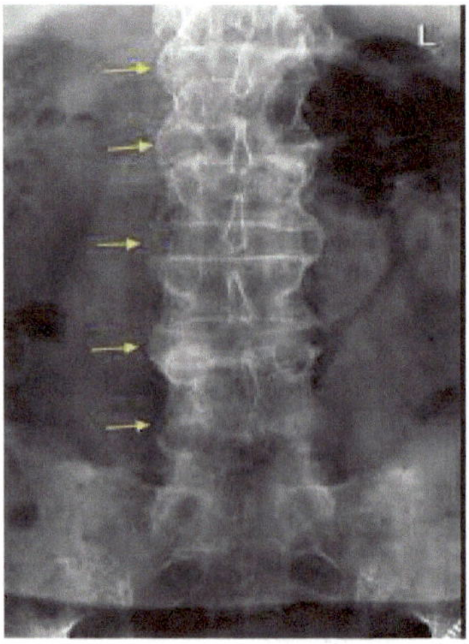

Answer: B i.e., Ankylosing spondylitis

70. **40 years old patient having arthritis of proximal interphalangeal joint and distal interphalangeal joint along with carpo-metacarpal joint of thumb and sparing of wrist and metacarpophalangeal joint. Most likely diagnosis is:**

(a) Rheumatoid arthritis
(b) Psoriatic arthropathy
(c) Osteoarthritis
(d) Pseudogout

Clinical presentation is suggestive of OA.

Osteoarthritis (OA) is the most common chronic joint condition. OA is also called wear-and-tear arthritis, degenerative arthritis, and degenerative joint disease.

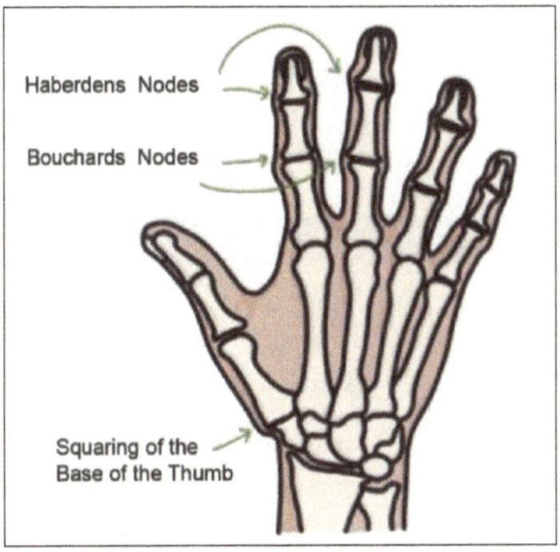

Answer: C i.e., Osteoarthritis

71. **A 35 years old male develops involvement of proximal interphalangeal joint, distal interphalangeal joint and metacarpophalangeal joints with sparing of the wrist and carpometacarpal joint. Most likely diagnosis:**

(a) Psoriatic arthropathy (b) Osteoarthritis

(c) Rheumatoid arthritis (d) Pseudogout

Clinical presentation is suggestive of psoriatic arthropathy.

Psoriatic arthritis is a chronic inflammatory arthritis that develops in at least 5% of patients with psoriasis.

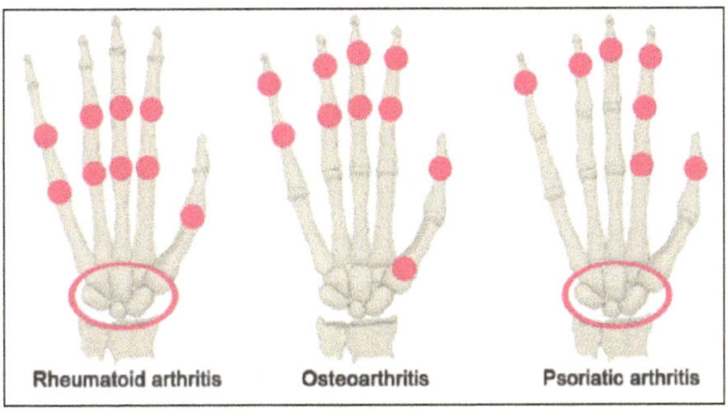

Answer: A i.e., Psoriatic arthropathy

72. An old lady presented with long standing arthritis of both hands and feet. X-ray feature which suggests rheumatoid arthritis, rather than seronegative spondyloarthropathies is:

(a) Loss of joint space (b) Peri-articular erosions

(c) Osteophytes (d) Periosteal reaction

RA is a chronic disease that causes joint pain, stiffness, swelling and decreased movement of the joints. Small joints in the hands and feet are most commonly affected.

Table 1: 1987 ACR Classification criteria for RA	
Criteria	1. Morning stiffness (at least one hour) 2. Arthritis in three or more joint areas 3. Arthritis of hand joints (≥ 1 swollen joints) 4. Symmetric arthritis 5. Rheumatoid nodules 6. Serum RF 7. Radiographic changes (erosions) on X-rays of hands
Applicable for	All arthritis patients
Results in	Classification of RA (yes/no)
Positive in case	Four of the seven criteria must be present. Criteria one through four must have been present for at least six weeks.

Answer: B i.e., Peri-articular erosions

73. A diabetic patient develops swelling of the knee joint, associated with sclerosis without deformity. Loose bodies are seen on aspiration. Most likely diagnosis:

(a) Neuropathic joint (b) Non-specific synovitis

(c) Osteoarthritis (d) Septic arthritis of knee

Clinical presentation is suggestive of neuropathic/ Charcot's joint.

Neuropathic arthropathy (Charcot joint) can be defined as bone and joint changes that occur secondary to loss of sensation and is most often associated with diabetes, syphilis, syringomyelia, spina bifida, traumatic spinal cord injury, and leprosy.

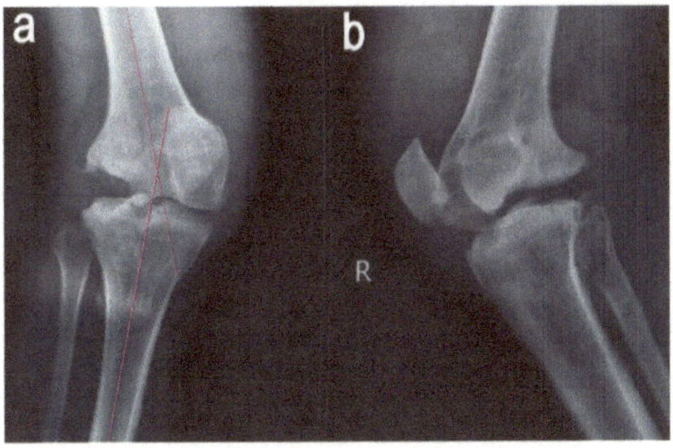

Answer: A i.e., Neuropathic joint

74. **A 60 years old man with diabetes mellitus presents with painless, swollen right ankle joint. Radiographs of the ankle show destroyed joint with large number of loose bodies. Most likely diagnosis:**

(a) Charcot's joint (b) Clutton's joint

(c) Osteoarthritis (d) Rheumatoid arthritis

Clinical presentation is suggestive of neuropathic/ Charcot's joint

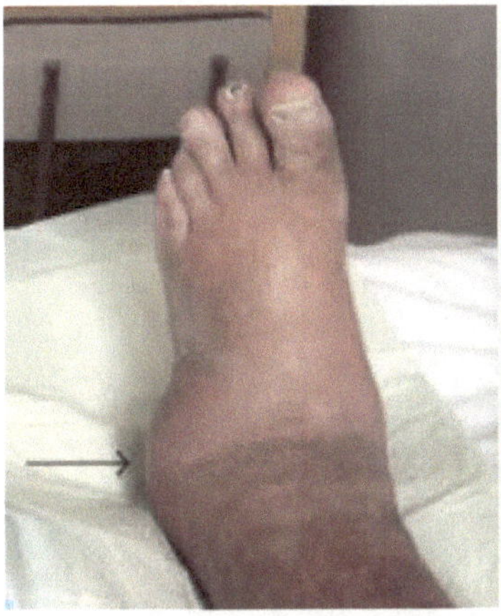

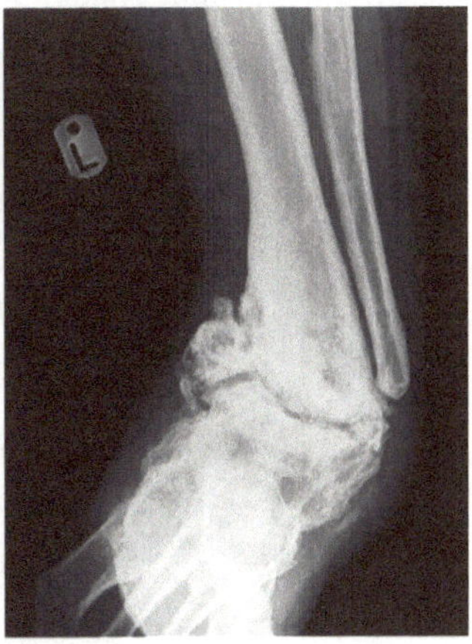

Answer: A i.e., Charcot's joint

75. **A lady presents with right knee swelling. Aspiration was done in which CPPD crystals were obtained. Likely diagnosis:**

(a) Osteoarthritis (b) Rheumatoid arthritis

(c) Gout (d) Pseudogout

Clinical presentation is suggestive of pseudogout.

Pseudogout is similar to gout but is generally less painful. It is caused by calcium pyrophosphate (CPP) crystals in the joints.

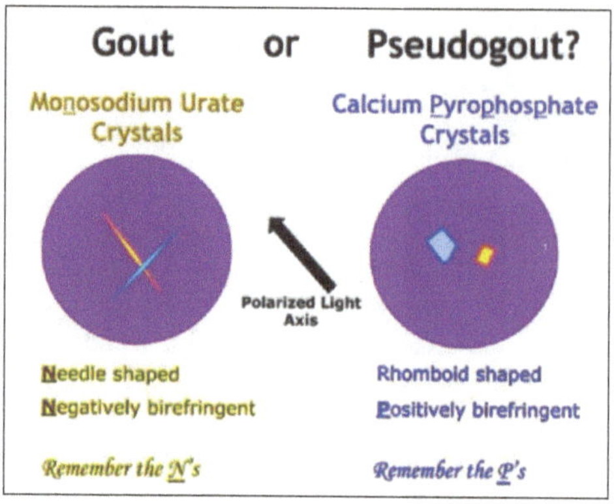

Answer: D i.e., Pseudogout

76. **A 65 years old man with history of back pain for 3 months. ESR is raised. On examination, marked stiffness and mild restriction of chest movements is found. On X-ray, syndesmophytes were present in vertebrae. Most likely diagnosis:**

(a) Ankylosing spondylitis

(b) Degenerative osteoarthritis of spine

(c) Lumbar canal stenosis

(d) Rheumatoid arthritis

Clinical presentation is suggestive of AS

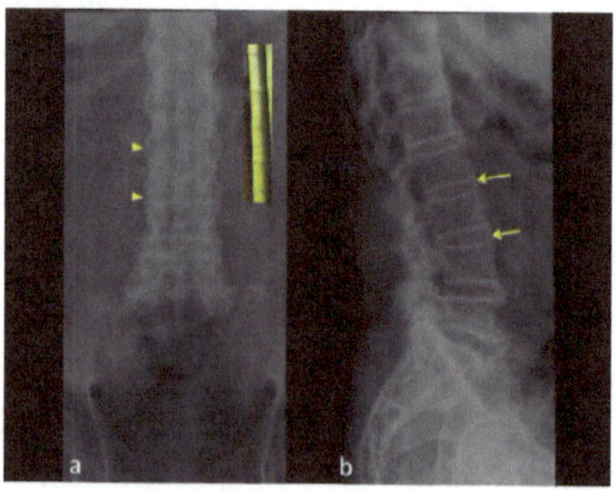

Answer: A i.e., Ankylosing spondylitis

77. **A 68 years old man came with pain and swelling of the right knee. Grade II osteoarthritis changes were found on investigation. Further management:**

(a) Arthroscopic washout (b) High tibial osteotomy

(c) Total knee replacement (d) Conservative

Grade II OA can be managed conservatively.

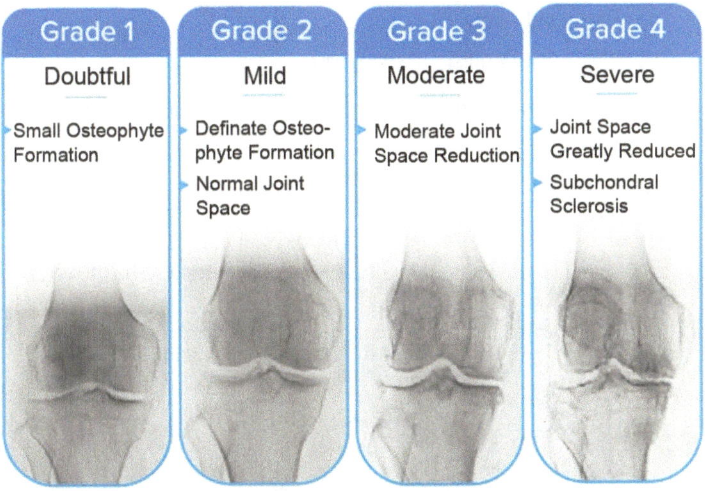

Answer: D i.e., Conservative

78. A newborn child presents with inverted foot and the dorsum of the foot cannot touch the anterior tibia. Most likely diagnosis:

(a) Congenital vertical talus (b) Arthrogryposis multiplex

(c) CTEV (d) Flat foot

Clinical presentation is suggestive of clubfoot/ CTEV.

Clubfoot is a deformity in which an infant›s foot is turned inward, often so severely that the bottom of the foot faces sideways or even upward.

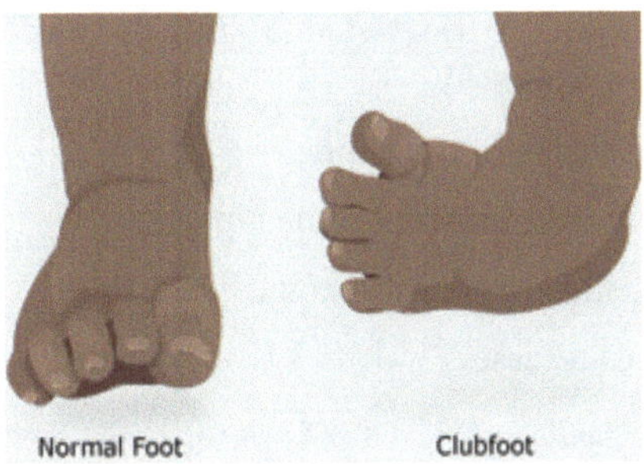

Answer: C i.e., CTEV

79. A 11-years old, 70 kg child presents with limitation of abduction and internal rotation. There is tender ness in Scarpa's (femoral) triangle. On flexing the hip, the limb is abducted. Most likely diagnosis:

(a) Perthes disease

(b) Slipped capital femoral epiphysis

(c) Observation hip

(d) Tuberculosis hip

Clinical presentation is suggestive of SCFE.

Slipped Capital Femoral Epiphysis refer to a fracture through the growth plate (physis), which results in slippage of the overlying end of the femur (metaphysis).

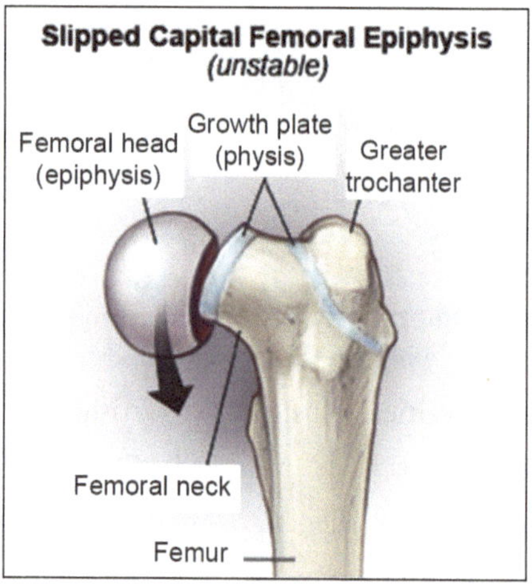

Answer: B i.e., Slipped capital femoral epiphysis

80. A 10 years old male with pain in the left hip and limping on examination, has restricted abduction and internal rotation. Most likely diagnosis:

(a) Septic arthritis of the hip

(b) Tuberculous arthritis of the hip

(c) Congenital dislocation of the hip

(d) Perthes disease

Clinical presentation is suggestive of Perthe's disease.

Legg–Calvé–Perthes disease (LCPD) is a childhood hip disorder initiated by a disruption of blood flow to the head of the femur.

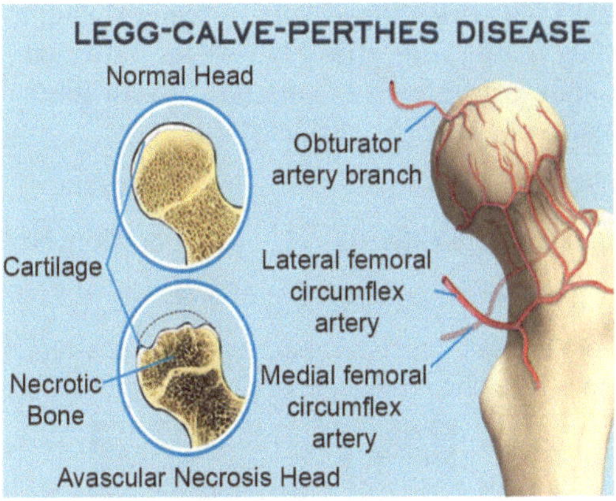

Answer: D i.e., Perthes disease

81. **A 2 years old male child has been limping ever since he has started walking. There is no pain. Examination reveals a short right lower limb with limited abduction at the hip. The Trendelenburg sign is positive however telescopy is absent. Most likely diagnosis:**

(a) Congenital dislocation of the hip

(b) Congenital coxa vara

(c) Perthe's disease

(d) Slipped capital femoral epiphysis

Clinical presentation is suggestive of congenital coxa vara.

Congenital — Coxa vara is a deformity of the hip, whereby the angle between the head and the shaft of the femur is reduced to less than 120 degrees.

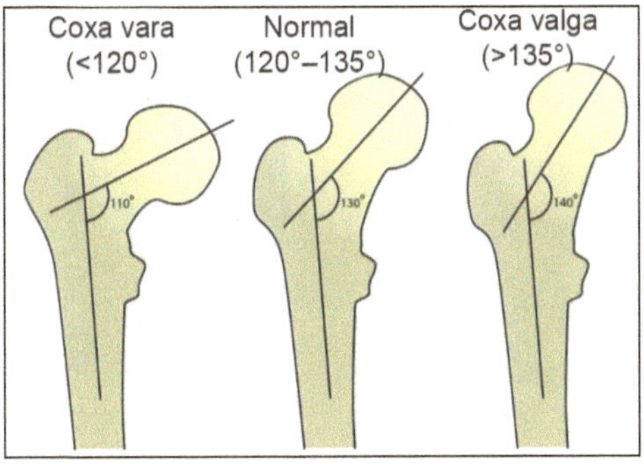

Answer: B i.e., Congenital coxa vara

82. A 15-years old with slipped capital femoral epiphysis develops increasing pain and stiffness in the affected hip. Serial X-rays shows progressive reduction in the joint space. What complication has the patient developed:

(a) Avascular necrosis (b) Coxa vara

(c) Secondary osteoarthritis (d) Chondrolysis

Clinical presentation is suggestive of AVN.

Avascular necrosis (AVN), also known as osteonecrosis, is a condition where bone tissue dies due to lack of blood supply.

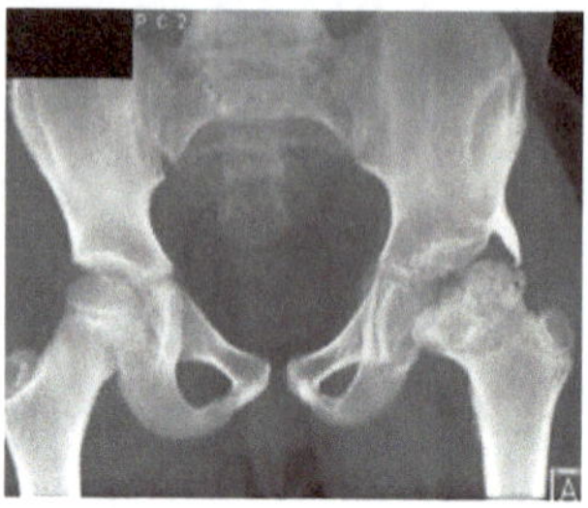

Answer: A i.e., Avascular necrosis

83. A 7 years old young boy, had fracture of lateral condyle of the femur. He developed malunion as the fracture was not reduced anatomically. Malunion will produce which deformity:

(a) Genu valgum (b) Genu varum

(c) Genu recurvatum (d) Wind swept deformity

Clinical presentation is suggestive of genu valgum.

Genu valgum, commonly called "knock-knee", is a condition in which the knees angle in and touch each other when the legs are straightened.

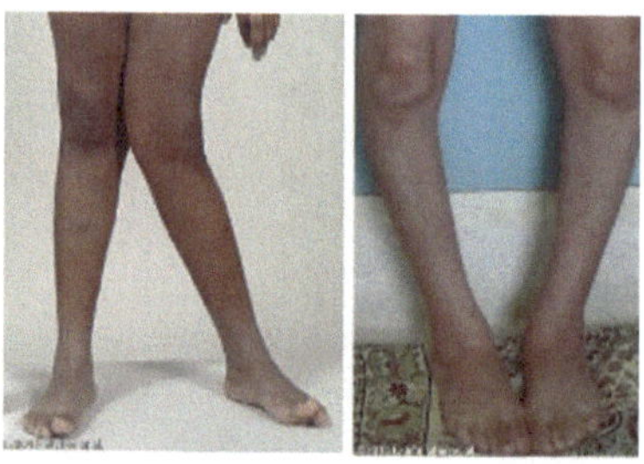

Genu Valgum "Knock-Knee" **Genu Varum** "Bow-legged"

Answer: A i.e., Genu valgum

84. A six years old boy presents with a painful limp. Clinical examination reveals tenderness in the femoral triangle and some limitation of hip movements. An X-ray was done which was normal. Next course of action:

(a) Wait and watch

(b) Ultrasonography

(c) Aspiration

(d) MRI scan

Clinical presentation is suggestive of transient synovitis of the hip/ observation hip.

Transient synovitis of the hip refers to a self-limiting acute inflammatory condition affecting the synovial lining of the hip.

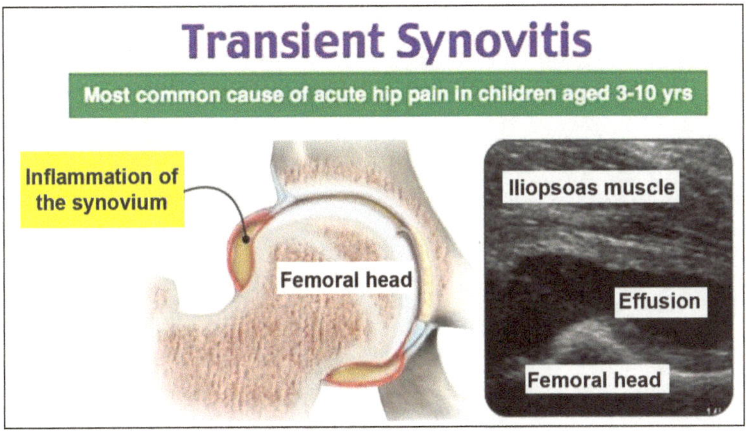

Answer: A i.e., Wait and watch

85. A 14-years old boy with 78 kg weight and hypothyroidism developed sudden onset of severe pain and tenderness on left hip as a result of minor fall. Most likely diagnosis:

(a) Fracture neck of femur

(b) Slipped capital femoral epiphysis

(c) Perthes disease

(d) Hip dislocation

Clinical presentation is suggestive of SCFE

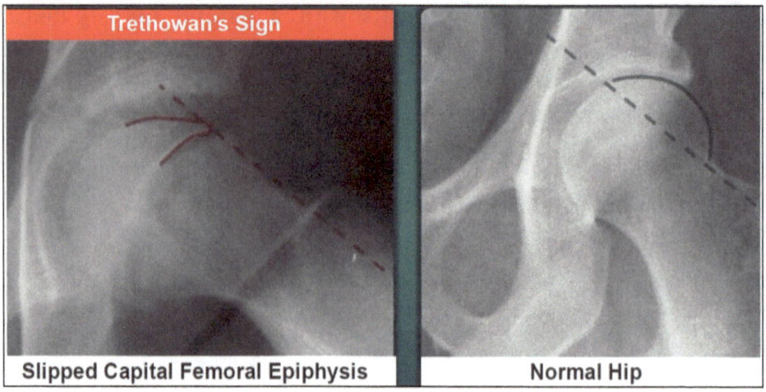

Answer: B i.e., Slipped capital femoral epiphysis

MCQs POINTS (One-liners)

No.	*Question*	*Answer*
1	Diagnosis of acute osteomyelitis is always	*Clinical*
2	Myositis ossificans is commonly seen in which muscle:	*Brachialis*
3	Unexplained backache of long duration should be evalauated for :	*TB spine*
4	Jones fracture involves which bone	*Base of 5th metatarsal*
5	Number of phalanx in thumb	*2*
6	Card test check which muscle	*Palmar interossei*
7	Subperiosteal haemorrhages may be seen n	*Scurvy*
8	Which nerve can be injured while operating near triceps	*Radial*
9	Three point relationship in supracondylar fracture humerus is :	*Maintained*
10	Burst fracture usually denotes fractures of:	*Vertebrae*
11	Action of gluteus maximus :	*Extension of hip*
12	Which ligament prevents backfalling of trunk	*Ileo-femoral*
13	Radiation induced bony tumour :	*Osteosarcoma*
14	Epiphyses in greater trochanter of femur	*Traction*
15	Tom Smith arthritis involves which joint	*Hip*
16	Hip spica is used for managing fracture s of:	*Shaft femur in children*
17	Complication of Volkmann's ischemia is:	*Volkmann Ischaemic Contracture/ VIC*
18	Cloacae are	*Holes in bone through which sequestrum comes out*
19	Nerve supply of quadriceps femoris	*Femoral*
20	Bouchard's nodes are found in:	*Osteoarthritis (PIP joint)*
21	Anterolateral decompression surgery is done for:	*Tb spine*

22	Osteoclastoma commonly arises from which part of bone:	*Epiphyses*
23	MC site of Osteosarcoma:	*Metaphysis*
24	Earliest involvement in hematogenous osteomyelitis is seen around which joint:	*Knee*
25	MC malignant primary tumour of bone:	*Multiple myeloma*
26	Nightstick fracture involves ....bone:	*Ulna*
27	Cylindrical cast is used in fractures of:	*Patella*
28	Knuckle bender splint is used for...nerve palsy:	*Ulnar*
29	McMurrays osteotomy is employed for:	*Non-union fracture neck of femur*
30	Head Halter/ Crutchfield traction is given for injuries in:	*Cervical spine*
31	Positive book test/ Froment sign suggest injury to .... Nerve:	*Ulnar*
32	Pointing index is due to palsy of ... nerve:	*Median*
33	Nerve involved in Saturday night palsy:	*Radial*
34	Injury to medial epicondyle of humerus results in injury to...nerve:	*Ulnar*
35	Phalen test is positive in:	*Carpal tunnel syndrome*
36	Dinner fork deformity is associated with.... fracture:	*Colle's fracture*
37	Position of immobilization of hand in Colles cast:	*Pronation, palmar flexion, ulnar deviation*
38	Best view (of wrist) for detecting fractures of Scaphoid:	*Oblique*
39	Rupture of nerve fibres with intact nerve sheath is known as:	*Axonotmesis*
40	MC joint to dislocate in body:	*Shoulder*
41	Position of limb in posterior dislocation of hip joint:	*Flexion, adduction & internal rotation*
42	Position (deformities) of foot in CTEV:	*Equinus, varus & forefoot adduction*
43	Another term for housemaid's knee:	*Prepatellar bursitis*
44	Salter & Harris classification is used for classifying:	*Epiphyseal injuries (children)*
45	Cubitus varus is maunited fracture of:	*Supracondylar humerus*

46	MC primary malignant tumour of bone:	*Multiple myeloma*
47	DOC (drug of choice) for osteoid osteoma:	*NSAID*
48	MC region of bone, involved in acute osteomyelitis:	*Metaphysis*
49	Cold abscess formation is suggestive of:	*Spinal TB*
50	Serum levels of calcium, phosphate, alkaline phosphatase & PTH in rickets:	*Low, low, high & high*
51	Pointing finger is due to injury to:	*Median nerve*
52	Looser's zone is characteristics of:	*Osteomalacia*
53	Lateral epicondyle fracture lately results in injury to:	*Ulnar nerve*
54	Tendo-Calcaneus lengthening is done in:	*Equinus deformity*
55	Lachman sign is positive in injury to:	*Anterior cruciate ligament/ ACL injury*
56	Sunray appearance is seen in:	*Osteosarcoma*
57	MC complication of fracture lower third of tibia:	*Delayed union/ non-union*
58	MC site of osteomyelitis:	*Lower end of femur/ upper end of tibia*
59	Myositis ossificans is commonly seen at the:	*Elbow joint*
60	Complete claw hand is seen in:	*Both Ulnar & median nerve injury*
61	Avulsion of terminal slip of extensor tendon to distal phalanx is known as:	*Mallet finger*
62	MC site of March fracture:	*2nd/ 3rd metatarsal*
63	Muscle tested in Froment's sign:	*Adductor pollicis*
64	Epiphyseal dysgenesis is a feature of:	*Hypo-thyroidism*
65	MC cause of tardy ulnar nerve palsy:	*Fracture lateral humeral condyle*
66	MC cause of neuropathic joints:	*Diabetes*
67	Monteggia fracture is:	*Fracture proximal third ulna with dislocation of superior radio-ulnar joint*
68	Nerve MC involved in fracture surgical neck of humerus:	*Axillary nerve*
69	Epiphyseal widening is a radiological sign of:	*Rickets*
70	Soap bubble appearance is seen in:	*Osteoclastoma/ Giant cell tumour*
71	Von Rosen splint is used in the management of:	*DDH/ CDH*

72	MC cause of posterior dislocation of hip joint:	*Dashboard injury (car)*
73	Rail-Road injury is:	*Concussion of spinal cord*
74	Prominent sign of Volkmann's ischemia is:	*Pain on passive extension*
75	Sequestrum is:	*Dead piece of bone, lying within the infected granulation tissue*
76	Linear striations are typically seen in:	*Vertebral hemangioma*
77	Heberden's nodes are found in:	*Osteoarthritis (DIP joint)*
78	Bankart's lesion involves:	*Glenoidal labrum*
79	Osteoclastoma commonly arises from which part of bone:	*Epiphyses*
80	MC site of Osteosarcoma:	*Metaphysis*
81	Earliest site of bone involvement in hematogenous osteomyelitis is seen in metaphysis because of:	*Hair-pin arrangement of vessels*
82	MC malignant tumour of bone:	*Secondaries*
83	Arthritis mutilans is seen in:	*Psoriasis*
84	Tension band wiring/ TBW is done for fractures of:	*Olecranon & patella*
85	Pott's fracture is:	*Bimalleolar fracture*
86	MC region of Pott's spine:	*Dorso-lumbar*
87	MC complication of trochnateric/ extracapsular fracture neck of femur:	*Mal-union*
88	Crutch palsy involves:	*Radial nerve*
89	Wrist drop is a manifestation of palsy of:	*Radial nerve*
90	Flexion at metacarpophalangeal joint & extension at interphalangeal joint is an action of which muscles:	*Lumbricals*
91	Ideal time for management of CTEV:	*Soon after the birth*
92	Tenderness in anatomical snuff box, after a history of fall on outstretched hand signifies fracture of:	*Scaphoid*
93	Clutton's joint is seen in:	*Congenital syphilis*
94	MC bone to fracture in childhood:	*Supracondylar humerus/ lower third humerus*

95	MC bone to fracture during birth:	*Clavicle*
96	MC type of shoulder dislocation:	*Anterior*
97	MC type of hip dislocation:	*Posterior*
98	MC bony tumour:	*Secondaries*
99	Hip joint TB heals by:	*Fibrous ankylosis*
100	Triple arthrodesis involves fusion of:	*Subtalar, talo-navicular & calcaneo-cuboid joints*
101	Charlie chaplin gait is seen in	*Tibial torsion*
102	Cozens test is done for	*Tennis elbow*
103	Osteochondritis of the capitulum (humerus) is known as	*Panners disease*
104	Avascular necrosis of head of femur occurs commonly at which region	*Subcapital*
105	Forced inversion in plantar flexed foot injuries result in damage to which ligament	*Talofibular*
106	Triple deformity of knee includes	*Flexion, posterior subluxation & external rotation*
107	Non-traumatic amputations can be seen in	*Leprosy, sickle cell anemia*
108	Salmonella osteomyelitis is MC in which condition	*Sickle cell anemia*
109	Austin Moore/AM prosthesis is used for which joint	*Hip*
110	Long axis of tibia and fibula moves lateral to the long axis of femur. This is known as	*Genu valgum*
111	Meralgia paresthetica involves which nerve	*Lateral cutaneous nerve of thigh*
112	Hand appearance in ulnar nerve injury	*Claw hand*
113	Rate of regeneration of nerves	*1 mm/day*
114	Ideal treatment of CTEV	*Corrective manipulation and serial casting (Ponseti technique)*
115	Early CTEV (less than 1 month old child) is best managed by	*Manipulation by mother*
116	Shepherd crook deformity is seen in	*Fibrous dysplasia*
117	Marble bone disease is also known as	*Osteopetrosis*

118	Characteristic sub-periosteal bone resorption in hyperparathyroidism is best seen in which bone	*Middle phalanx (radial side)*
119	In renal dystrophy, skeletal abnormality is most commonly due to	*Hyper-phosphataemia*
120	Triple arthrodesis is done for which condition	*CTEV*
121	Indication of surgical compartment release in compartment syndrome in any compartment is absolute pressure greater than	*30 mm Hg*
122	Pseudoflexion deformity at hip is commonly seen in	*Ilio-psoas abscess*
123	Management of congenital pseudo-arthrosis of tibia	*Vascularized fibular graft*
124	Nerve closely realted to shoulder joint capsule	*Axillary*
125	Dupuytrens contracture most often involves which finger	*Ring finger*
126	Lower limb is in abduction, external rotation & flexion. Diagnosis	*Anterior dislocation hip*
127	Extremely low birth weight is defined as weight of an infant below:	*1 kg*
128	Apprehension sign is positive for:	*Shoulder dislocation (recurrent)*
129	McMurrays test are done to detect:	*Meniscal injury knee*
130	Thomas test is done to detect which deformity at hip	*Fixed flexion deformity at hip*
131	Boxers fracture involves ....bone:	*5th metacarpal*
132	Cylindrical cast is used in fractures of:	*Patella*
133	Knuckle bender splint is used for...nerve palsy:	*Ulnar*
134	McMurrays osteotomy is employed for:	*Non-union fracture neck of femur*
135	Gallow traction is given for fractures of which bone:	*Femur*
136	Positive book test suggest paralysis of ..... muscle:	*Adductor pollicis*
137	Pointing index is due to palsy of ... muscle:	*FDS, FDP (lateral half)*
138	Nerve involved in Saturday night palsy:	*Radial*
139	Injury to lateral epicondyle of humerus results in injury to... nerve:	*Ulnar*
140	Tingling & numbness in lateral three and a half digits suggest the diagnosis of	*Carpal tunnel syndrome*

141	Upper limb fracture commonly associated with osteoporosis:	*Colle's fracture*
142	Position of immobilization of hand for fracture scaphoid:	*Glass holding position*
143	Best view (of wrist) for detecting fractures of Scaphoid:	*Oblique*
144	Neuropraxia is defined as	*Anatomical intact, physiological cessation of activity*
145	MC joint to re-dislocate in body:	*Shoulder*
146	Position of upper limb in Erb's palsy:	*Extension, adduction & medial rotation*
147	Triple arthrodesis in CTEV should be done after the age of	*Skeletal maturity (physis closure)*
148	Students elbow is	*Olecranon bursitis*
149	Thurston Holland sign is seen in	*Epiphyseal injuries (children)*
150	Brachial artery may be commonly involved in fracture of:	*Supracondylar humerus*
151	MC benign tumour of bone:	*Osteochondroma*
152	Location for osteoid osteoma:	*Compact bone*
153	MC diagnostic feature of chronic osteomyelitis:	*Discharge of bony spicules through sinus*
154	Gibbus is a feature of:	*Spinal TB*
155	Surgical management of volkmann's ischaemic contracture	*Maxpage operation*
156	Sunburst appearance is radiological finding of which tumour	*Osteosarcoma*
157	Management of posterior dislocation of hip	*Immediate reduction*
158	Champagne glass pelvis, on X-ray is suggestive of	*Achondroplasia*
159	Condition in which there is either anterior or posterior displacement of a vertebrae with respect to the vertebrae below	*Spondylo-listhesis*
160	Finkelstein test is done for which condition	*DeQuervain tenosynovitis*
161	Which muscle is chief extensor of knee joint	*Quadriceps femoris*
162	MC type of vertebral involvement in TB spine	*Paradiscal*
163	Injury to C5 & C6 nerve roots can lead to	*Erb's palsy*

164	Multiple fractures in a child without any healing suggest the diagnosis of	*Osteogenesis imperfecta*
165	Multiple fractures in a child in multiple stages of healing suggest the diagnosis of	*Battered baby syndrome*
166	MC facial bone to fracture	*Nasal*
167	Attitude of joints in Boutonniere deformity	*Flexion contracture of PIP, extension of DIP*
168	Gower sign is seen in	*Duchenne muscular dystrophy*
169	Which joint is spared in rheumatoid arthritis	*DIP/ distal interphalangeal joint*
170	Fracture neck of fibula may injure which nerve	*Common peroneal nerve*
171	Fracture proximal ulna with dislocation of proximal radio-ulnar joint is known as	*Monteggia fracture dislocation*
172	MC true benign bone tumour	*Osteoid osteoma*
173	Ocular finding in a case of ankylosing spondylitis	*Acute anterior uveitis*
174	Hill Sach's lesion is seen with recurrent dislocation of which joint	*Shoulder*
175	Scaphoid fracture clinically present as tenderness in which landmark	*Anatomical snuff box*
176	MC cause of sciatic nerve damage	*Iatrogenic (Intramuscular injections)*
177	IOC for congenital dislocation of hip in an infant	*USG*
178	Which ligament of foot is at fault in pes planus	*Spring ligament*
179	First sign of impending compartment syndrome	*Pain on passive stretch*
180	Charcot's joint is defined as	*Neuropathic joint*
181	MC site of fracture of mandible is	*Neck*
182	Related to nerve injuries, motor march is seen in which type	*Axonotmesis*
183	Age of presentation of Ewing sarcoma	*Second decade*
184	Function of anterior cruciate ligament	*Prevents anterior dislocation of tibia*
185	Kienbock disease is avascular necrosis of	*Lunate*
186	Stress fracture is commonly seen in	*Metatarsals*
187	Spina ventosa is known as	*TB Dactylitis*

188	Which nerve is commonly involved in anterior dislocation of shoulder	*Axillary*
189	IOC for avascular necrosis	*MRI*
190	Median nerve is commonly involved in fractures of	*Supracondylar humerus*
191	Brachial artery may be injured in	*Supracondylar fracture humerus*
192	HLA-B27 is associated with	*Ankylosing spondylitis*
193	Defective mineralization of osetoid is seen in	*Rickets*
194	Colle's fracture involves	*Distal radius*
195	Fracture neck of femur is also known as	*Intracapsular fracture femur*
196	Carpal tunnel syndrome is managed by	*Decompression surgery (release of flexor retinaculum)*
197	Faulty technique of intramuscular injection over deltoid can injure	*Axillary nerve*
198	Brachioradialis is supplied by	*Radial nerve*
199	Foot drop may be a manifestation of injury to which nerve	*Deep peroneal nerve*
200	Haversian canal is a histological feature of	*Diaphysis*
201	MC cause of acute osteomyelitis in sickle cell anemia	*Salmonella typhi*
202	Earliest radiological sign of TB spine	*Reduction of intervertebral disc space*
203	Premalignant condition for osteosarcoma	*Paget's disease*
204	Von-Rosen splint keeps the lower limb in which position	*Abducted and external rotated*
205	U cast is used for fractures of…	*Shaft of humerus*
206	Winging of scapula is due to involvement of which muscle	*Serratus anterior*
207	Bence Jones protein is seen in	*Multiple myeloma*
208	Ortolani test is done for	*Developmental dysplasia of hip*
209	Fracture 5th metacarpal is known as	*Boxer's fracture*
210	Boston brace is used for	*Scoliosis*
211	Adult counterpart of rickets	*Osteomalacia*
212	Amyloidosis may be a complication of	*Chronic osteomyelitis*
213	Most common type of elbow dislocation	*Posterior*

214	MC bone to be involved in Pott's disease:	*Vertebrae*
215	Bennet's fracture involve	*Base of first metacarpal*
216	Supinator is related to which nerve	*Posterior interosseus branch of Radial nerve*
217	Swan neck & Z-deformity of fingers is seen in which ...... arthritis	*Rheumatoid*
218	Common manifestation of Ankylosing spondylitis:	*Sacro-ilitis*
219	Backward slipping of one vertebrae over other is known as:	*Retro-listhesis*
220	Hawkin's sign is related to which fracture	*Neck of talus*
221	Nerve injured in posterior dislocation of hip:	*Sciatic*
222	Pain on passive stretching of fingers after injury may suggest the possibility of:	*Impending compartment syndrome*
223	Recurrent dislocation of patella occurs commonly on which side:	*Lateral*
224	Example of atavistic epiphyses	*Coracoid process*
225	Cubital tunnel syndrome is due to compression of which nerve:	*Ulnar nerve*
226	Tumour that usually stops growing in size with physeal closure:	*Exostosis/ osteo-chondroma*
227	MC bone sarcoma in children:	*Ewings sarcoma*
228	Nerve MC injured in maxillary fractures:	*Infraorbital nerve*
229	HLA antigen linked to anterior uveitis:	*HLA B27*
230	Tension band wiring principle:	*Distraction forces are converted into compressive forces*
231	MC fractured bone of face:	*Nasal*
232	Tarsal tunnel syndrome is due to compression of which nerve:	*Posterior tibial nerve*
233	Which type of infection usually results in bony ankylosis:	*TB of spine & pyogenic infection*
234	LeFort classification is used for fractures of which bone:	*Maxilla*
235	Potts puffy tumour is also known as:	*Chronic frontal osteomyelitis*
236	Tinel sign suggests ...... of nerve:	*Regeneration*

237	Around elbow, which epiphyses ossifies first:	*Capitulum*
238	Hill Sach lesion is seen in recurrent dislocation of which joint:	*Shoulder*
239	A young male presented with joint pain & backache. X-ray of the spine shows evidence of sacro-ilitis. Diagnosis	*Ankylosing spondylitis*
240	Most characteristically involved joint in Rheumatoid arthritis:	*Meta-carpophalngeal joint*
241	MC cause of multiple fractures in childhood:	*Osteogenesis imperfecta*
242	Ape thumb deformity is due to injury to which nerve:	*Median nerve*
243	Fracture of cervical vertebra one is known as	*Jefferson's fracture*
244	Medial half of flexor digitorum profundus is supplied by which nerve	*Ulnar*
245	Boxers muscle is:	*Serratus anterior*
246	Sun-ray appearance is suggestive of which bony tumour:	*Osteosarcoma*
247	Subperiosteal resorptions are seen in which metabolic disorder:	*Hyper-parathyroidism*
248	Nerve passing between two heads of pronator teres muscle	*Median nerve*
249	Boutoneirre's deformity is seen in:	*Rheumatoid arthritis*
250	'Pseudo-flexion deformity at hip is due to spasm of which muscle	*Ilio-psoas*
251	TB spine is also known as:	*Pott's disease*
252	Spindle shaped expansion of the bone in TB dactylitis is known as:	*Spina ventosa*
253	Oschgood Schlatter's disease is osteochondritis of:	*Tibial tubercle*
254	Nerve damaged in fracture supracondylar humerus:	*Median nerve (anterior interosseous branch)*
255	Claw hand is a manifestation of:	*Ulnar nerve (+ median nerve in complete clawing)*
256	Blow-out injuries with ptosis are characteristic of:	*Orbital injury*
257	Sausage digits are seen in:	*Psoriasis*
258	Loss of opposition is seen in:	*Median nerve injury*

259	Fracture neck of femur in an elderly is managed by:	*Hemi-replacement arthroplasty*
260	Shoulder joint is reinforced by which structure :	*Rotator cuff*
261	Cancellous bone is present in which part of bone	*Metaphysis*
262	Example of pressure epiphyses:	*Femoral head*
263	MC type of TB spine	*Paradiscal*
264	Oblique X-ray view is helpful for which fracture	*Scaphoid*
265	Splint used in ulnar nerve injury	*Knuckle bender splint*
266	Fat embolism is usually associated with fracture of	*Femur*
267	Fracture involving both malleoli is known as	*Pott's fracture*
268	McMurray test is done for injury to which structure	*Meniscus of knee*
269	Froment sign checks which muscle	*Adductor pollicis*
270	Card test checks which muscle	*Palmar interossei*
271	MC cause of death after total hip replacement	*Pulmonary thrombo-embolism*
272	Acute gouty arthritis is managed by	*Colchicine*
273	MC involved joint in pseudogout	*Knee*
274	Drug of choice for senile osteoporosis	*Estrogen*
275	Calcium & phosphorous level in osteoporosis	*Normal*
276	Paget's disease is associated with which cancer	*Osteosarcoma*
277	Osteoid osteoma is also known as	*Aspirin tumour*
278	Trident hand is seen in	*Achondro-plasia*
279	Brittle bone disease is	*Osteogenesis imperfecta*
280	Commonest pathology (of hip) in congenital dislocation of hip	*Shallow acetabulum*
281	MC cause of genu valgum in children	*Rickets*
282	Wind swept deformity is seen in	*Rickets*
283	Earliest radiological change in RA	*Periarticular osteopenia*
284	Joint spared in RA	*DIP*
285	Trendelenburg test checks which muscles	*Gluteus medius & Gluetus minimus*
286	Diagnostic sign of a fracture	*Crepitus*
287	Radiation induced bony tumour	*Osteosarcoma*
288	Location of giant cell tumour in bone	*Epiphysis*

289	MC bony tumour in hand	*Enchondroma*
290	Management of clavicle fracture	*Figure of 8 bandage*
291	Tinel sign is seen in	*Nerve regeneration*
292	MC type of shoulder dislocation	*Anterior subcoracoid*
293	MC involved bone in Paget's disease	*Pelvis*
294	Undertaker's fracture is involves which vertebrae	*C6-C7*
295	Age group affected in Perthe's disease	*4-8 years*
296	Investigation of choice for spinal TB	*MRI*
297	MC site of TB in body	*Vertebrae*
298	Trendleneberg test is positive in injury to which nerve	*Superior gluteal nerve*
299	Gait of a patient with bilateral CDH	*Waddling*
300	Winging of scapula is because of palsy of which muscle	*Serratus anterior*
301	Calcium levels in osteomalacia	*Low*
302	MC age group affected in acute osteomyelitis	*Second decade*
303	Age group affected in giant cell tumour	*20-40 years*
304	Aspirin is used in relieving pain of which tumour	*Osteoid osteoma*
305	MC nerve injured in posterior dislocation of hip joint	*Sciatic*
306	In a case of partial amputation with heavy contamination, first step in management should be	*Wound irrigation & debridement*
307	Immediate treatment of patient with multiple fracture and fluid loss is best done by	*Ringer lactate*
308	Risser Localiser cast is used in the management of	*Idiopathic scoliosis*
309	Last step in healing of a fracture is	*Modelling*
310	Neuropraxia is condition is characterized by	*Physiological block*
311	Which structure is fixed first during re-implantation of an amputated digit	*Bone*
312	Bicipital grove is present in which bone	*Humerus*
313	Indication for surgical compartment release in compartment syndrome, if the absolute pressure is greater than	*30 mm Hg*
314	Milkman's fracture is also known as	*Pseudofracture*
315	Circumferential growth of bone occurs because of	*Periosteum*

316	Periosteum is attached to bone by	*Sharpe's fibres*
317	Marker of new bone formation	*Alkaline phosphatase*
318	LeFort classification is used for	*Fractures of maxilla*
319	Thurston-Holland sign is seen in Salter-Harris	*Type II epiphyseal injuries*
320	Another term for extra-trochanteric fractures of femur	*Extra-capsular fracture of femur*
321	Displacement of distal fragment in Colle's fracture	*Dorsal & lateral*
322	Commonest cause of compartment syndrome	*Fractures*
323	Action of intramedullary K-nail	*3 point fixation*
324	In flap method of amputation, which structure is kept shorter than the level of amputation	*Bone*
325	MC site of fracture mandible	*Neck of condyle*
326	Cause of atonic bladder	*Injury to sacral plexus*
327	Bechterew disease is also known as	*Ankylosing spondylitis*
328	Tripod fracture is seen in	*Zygomatic bone*
329	MC site of disc herniation	*L4-L5*
330	Osteopetrosis is because of defective	*Osteoclasts*
331	Pointing finger is due to injury to:	*Median nerve*
332	Cold abscess is related to which clinical condition	*TB spine*
333	Garden's classification is used for classifying fracture sof	*Neck of femur*
334	Tendo-Calcaneus lengthening is done in:	*Equinus deformity*
335	Anterior drawer test is positive in injury to:	*Anterior cruciate ligament injury*
336	Sunray appearance is seen in:	*Osteosarcoma*
337	MC complication of fracture lower third of tibia:	*Delayed union/ non-union*
338	MC site of osteomyelitis:	*Lower end of femur/ upper end of tibia*
339	Myositis ossificans is commonly seen at the:	*Elbow joint*
340	Complete claw hand is seen in:	*Both Ulnar & median nerve injury*
341	Avulsion of terminal slip of extensor tendon to distal phalanx is known as:	*Mallet finger*

342	A bone is weakened by some disease and hence fractures even with minor trauma. This is known as :	*Pathological fracture*
343	Muscle tested in Froment's sign:	*Adductor pollicis*
344	Epiphyseal dysgenesis is a feature of:	*Hypo-thyroidism*
345	In a suspected case of fracture, what should be done at the earliest	*Immobilization*
346	MC cause of neuropathic joints:	*Diabetes*
347	Monteggia fracture is defined as :	*Fracture proximal third ulna with dislocation of superior radio-ulnar joint*
348	Nerve MC involved in fracture surgical neck of humerus:	*Axillary nerve*
349	Epiphyseal widening is a radiological sign of:	*Rickets*
350	Soap bubble appearance is seen in:	*Osteoclastoma/ Giant cell tumour*
351	Von Rosen splint is used in the management of:	*DDH/ CDH*
352	Attitude of limb in case of TB hip synovitis stage	*Flexion, abduction & external rotation*
353	Rail-Road injury is:	*Concussion of spinal cord*
354	Bumper fracture involves	*Tibial condyle*
355	Sequestrum appearance on X-rays	*Radiodense*
356	Characteristic subperiosteal resorption in hyperparathyroidism is best seen in which bone	*Radial border of middle phalanx*
357	MC site of malignant spine compression	*Thoracic*
358	Progression of congenital scoliosis is LEAST likely in which vertebral anomaly	*Block vertebrae*
359	A patient involved in RTA presents with quadripareisis, sphincter disturbances, sensory level upto the upper border of sternum and a respiratory rate of 35/ minute. Most likely level of lesion is	*C4-C5*
360	Autologous bone graft is commonly taken from	*Iliac crest*
361	Motorcyclist's fracture is	*The base of skull break in two halves left lateral and right lateral*
362	MC force involved in fracture of the spine is	*Flexion*

363	Mechanism of violence in burst fracture of the spine	*Compression violence*
364	Rugger Jersey spine is seen in	*Renal osteodystrophy*
365	Shoulder sicca is	*TB of shoulder joint*
366	A young man met with an accident and had mild quadripareisis. His lateral X-ray of cervical spine revealed C5-C6 fracture dislocation. Best line of management of such a case	*Cervical traction followed by instrument fixation*
367	Investigation of choice in suspected Perthe's disease	*MRI*
368	Superiosteal resorption intermingled with sclerotic radiopaque areas in skull is seen in	*Hyperparathyroidism*
369	In actinomycosis of the spine, the abscess usually erodes	*Towards the skin*
370	A classical expansive lytic lesion in the transverse process of a vertebrae is seen in	*Aneurysmal bone cyst*
371	A 9 year old child presents with scoliosis, hairy tuft in the skin at the back & neurological deficit. Plain X-ray reveal multiple vertebral anomalies and vertical bony spur overlying lumbar spine on AP view. Most probable diagnosis	*Diastometamyelia*
372	In a patient with head injury, unexplained hypotension warrants evaluation of which vertebral region	*Thoracic*
373	MC site of actinomycosis	*Mandible*
374	Jefferson's fracture involves which vertebrae	*C1*
375	Most important single investigation on lumbar disc prolpase is	*MRI*
376	Compression fracture is commonest in which vertebral spine	*Lower thoracic spine*
377	Deafnes in Pendred syndrome is due to	*Narrowing of foramina of skull*
378	In fracture calcaneum, which other injuries should be ruled out	*Fracture spine*
379	Ankylosis in TB hip joint	*Fibrous*
380	Mortar & pestle appearance is seen in	*TB hip*
381	Tinel sign is done clinically to check:	*Nerve regeneration*
382	Triple deformity of knee is a feature of:	*TB knee*
383	MC cause of Charcot's joints:	*Diabetes*
384	Damage to the radial nerve in the spiral grove spares:	*Long head of triceps*

385	Meralgia paresthetica involves:	*Lateral cutaneous nerve of thigh*
386	Cubitus varus is commonly due to:	*Malunited supracondylar fracture of humerus*
387	Management of Smith's fracture is:	*Above elbow cast with forearm in supination*
388	Ortolani's test is done for:	*CDH/ DDH*
389	Treatment of choice for one week old fracture neck femur at 65 years age is:	*Hemi-replacement arthroplasty*
390	MC benign tumour of bone:	*Osteochondroma*
391	Solitary bone cyst is most common in the:	*Upper end of humerus*
392	Erosion of bone is NOT seen in:	*SLE*
393	True regarding phantom limb:	*Follows amputation*
394	The commonest complication of Colle's fracture is:	*Stiffness of fingers*
395	Injury to the ulnar nerve at the wrist causes paralysis of:	*Adduction of thumb*
396	Supinator muscle is related to which nerve :	*Posterior interosseus nerve*
397	Joint commonly involved in Osteochondritis dessicans:	*Knee joint*
398	Painless effusion in joint in congenital syphilis is called:	*Clutton's joint*
399	In rheumatoid arthritis, pathology starts in which structure of joint:	*Synovium*
400	Treatment of choice for Paget's disease of the bone is:	*Calcitonin*
401	Gibbus is seen in which condition :	*TB spine*
402	Musculocutaenous nerve supplies which muscles :	*Biceps, brachialis and coracobrachialis*
403	Regiment badge sig is seen in injury to:	*Axillary nerve*
404	Most common type of supracondylar fracture is:	*Extension type*
405	NOT a complication of Colle's fracture:	*Non-union*
406	Most common site of fracture neck femur that cause avascular necrosis is:	*Subcapital*
407	Treatment of choice in fracture neck femur in a 40 year old male presenting after 2 days is:	*Closed reduction & internal fixation by cancellous screws*

408	Intramedullary 'K' nail is used for managing fractures of :	*Femoral shaft*
409	Which type of injury causes more damage to the semilunar cartilage in the knee:	*Rotation on a flexed knee*
410	MC true benign bone tumour:	*Osteoid osteoma*
411	Triple arthrodesis is done for	*Neglected CTEV*
412	Postero-medial Soft Tissue Release is done in CTEV after the age of	*2 years*
413	Most common complication of Colle's fracture is:	*Stiffness of fingers*
414	Open reduction & internal fixation is needed for which fractures in childhood:	*Lateral humeral condyle*
415	Tennis elbow is characterized by:	*Tendonitis of common extensor origin*
416	Union is facilitated by	*Hematoma*
417	Most common site of scaphoid fracture is	*Waist*
418	First symptom in tuberculous cord compression is	*Spasticity*
419	Most common Charcoat's joints involved in diabetes mellitus are those of	*Foot*
420	Characteristic crystals in pseudogout are	*Calcium pyrophosphate*
421	Atrophy of thenar area is due to injury to	*Median nerve*
422	Hollowing of dorsum of hand is noticed in palsy of	*Ulnar nerve*
423	No-mens land is related to injury of	*Tendons of hand*
424	Technique of casting in CTEV	*Ponseti*
425	Skyline view is employed for which joint	*Knee*
426	Sunray appearance is because of	*Calcification along the blood vessels*
427	Union in spiral fractures is good because of	*More surface area*
428	Region of bone affected in acute osteomyelitis in children	*Metaphysis*
429	Lift-off test is done for which muscle	*Subscapularis*
430	Gamekeeper thumb is injury to	*Ulnar collateral ligament*
431	Most vascular zone in a bone	*Metaphysis*
432	Attitude of DIP/ distal interphalangeal joint in Boutonierre deformity	*Extended*
433	Inferior dislocation of shoulder joint is known as	*Luxatio erecta*

434	Froment sign suggest injury to which nerve	*Ulnar nerve*
435	Action of extensor carpi radialis longus	*Extension & radial deviation of wrist*
436	Which region of spine is commonly affected in rheumatoid arthritis	*Cervical spine*
437	Fixed flexion deformity at hip is detected by which test	*Thomas test*
438	Chondrosarcoma commonly occurs at	*Pelvis*
439	Nodes on DIP in osteoarthritis	*Heberden's nodes*
440	Gait in bilateral developmental dysplasia of hip	*Waddling*
441	In fracture supracondylar humerus, the three point relationship is	*Maintained*
442	Parathyroid hormone acts on which cells	*Osteoblasts*
443	Bacteria commonly causing acute osteomyelitis	*Staphylococcus aureus*
444	Muscle used as a substitute for wrist extensors in a case with radial nerve palsy	*Pronator teres*
445	In trigger finger, pathology is at which joint	*Metacarpophalangeal joint*
446	Knee deformity which may be seen in rheumatoid arthritis	*Wind-swept deformity*
447	L4,L5 prolapsed intervertebral disc can give a positive	*Trendlenburg test*
448	Gap non-union can be managed by	*Bone transport*
449	Hamilton ruler test is positive in	*Anterior shoulder dislocation*
450	Trendlenburg test is positive in injury to which nerve	*Superior gluteal nerve*
451	Clinical manifestation of deep peroneal nerve injury	*Foot drop*
452	Jersey finger is due to avulsion injury of which tendon	*Flexor digitorum profundus*
453	High stepping gait is a feature of	*Foot drop*
454	Maximum weight given in skin traction	*4-5 kgs*
455	Most common site of fracture, which leads to fat embolism	*Fracture shaft of femur*
456	Common site of enchondroma	*Phalanges*
457	Wandering acetabulum is seen in	*TB of hip*
458	Pathognomonic feature of rheumatoid arthritis	*Rheumatoid nodule*

459	Another term for Paget's disease of bone	***Osteitis deformans***
460	Short 4th and 5th metacarpal is seen in	***Pseudo-hypo-parathyroidism***
461	Most common cause of genu valgum in children	***Rickets***
462	Trauma to surgical neck of humerus can paralyze	***Axillary nerve***